Yoga – Anticolonial Philosophy

With Best Wishes

of related interest

Ayurveda in Yoga Teaching
A Handbook for Enriching Āsana, Prāṇāyāma, Meditation and Yoga Nidrā
Tarik Dervish
Illustrations by Masha Pimas
ISBN 978 1 78775 595 6
eISBN 978 1 78775 596 3

The Yoga Teacher's Survival Guide
Social Justice, Science, Politics, and Power
Edited by Theo Wildcroft and Harriet McAtee
Foreword by Matthew Remski
ISBN 978 1 80501 166 8
eISBN 978 1 80501 167 5

YOGA – ANTICOLONIAL PHILOSOPHY

An Action-Focused Guide to Practice

SHYAM RANGANATHAN

SINGING DRAGON
LONDON AND PHILADELPHIA

First published in Great Britain in 2024 by Singing Dragon,
an imprint of Jessica Kingsley Publishers
Part of John Murray Press

1

Front cover image source: Shutterstock® and Deposit Photos.

A CIP catalogue record for this title is available from the
British Library and the Library of Congress

ISBN 978 1 83997 876 0
eISBN 978 1 83997 877 7

Printed and bound in the United States by Integrated Books International

Jessica Kingsley Publishers' policy is to use papers that are natural, renewable and recyclable products and made from wood grown in sustainable forests. The logging and manufacturing processes are expected to conform to the environmental regulations of the country of origin.

Singing Dragon
Carmelite House
50 Victoria Embankment
London EC4Y 0DZ

www.singingdragon.com

John Murray Press
Part of Hodder & Stoughton Limited
An Hachette UK Company

For my family

Contents

Preface

I am used to writing academic tracts. As a university teacher, I am also used to teaching students who are absolute beginners with no background in all that is being taught. This book is a blend of these two exercises. Perhaps the most surprising finding of my teaching career is that the one text that has the most profound impact on my students is the *Yoga Sūtra*. Unlike typical Yoga gurus, as a Philosophy professor, I'm not a one-trick pony. I teach my students the canon from the Western tradition and whatever Asian philosophy I can fit into the syllabus. But the *Yoga Sūtra* is by far the most impactful text that I can share. And that pedagogical exercise of teaching Yoga to my Philosophy students has deepened my appreciation for its importance in life.

When I entered Yogaland as a public philosopher and scholar willing to teach and share my practice, I was surprised at the position of many South Asian teachers who fast became my friends. Many of them were highly accomplished individuals who were annoyed that Yoga spaces and conferences gave deference to non-South Asians. These friends of mine insisted that this constituted not only discrimination against South Asian teachers but also disinformation, which could be corrected by prioritizing South Asian teachers. My initial reaction was disagreement for two reasons. First, being South Asian does not confirm any special knowledge about Yoga. Indeed, in ancient times, this was widely attested to by the expectation that in order to learn Philosophy and Yoga, one typically had to leave one's home life and seek out unusual life experiences and teachers to engage in the personal experimentation necessary to learn about Yoga. Yoga, a Devotion to Sovereignty, is not anything that happens passively as a result of upbringing. You have to work at it. So on the basis of the ancient South Asian tradition alone, I found this idea that we need more

South Asian representation false, as mere representation would do nothing. Second, I already knew that the idea that knowledge is a cultural artefact was Aristotelian, Platonic, and an important part of the *West*'s colonial heritage. By making knowledge a matter of culture and upbringing, the *West* confuses its own culture with the frame of knowledge. South Asians helping themselves to this Aristotelian and Platonic idea were not actually indigenizing or decolonizing Yoga: they were acting out their own *West*-ern colonization and colonizing Yoga. This observation generalizes. Often people from colonized traditions tired of *W*estern enculturation want to replace it with the enculturation of the colonized tradition *as though* that is decolonization. But the idea that enculturation is pedagogy is as *W*estern as it gets and is an essential part of the mechanism of any colonial tradition.

What I did not really appreciate was the extent to which my South Asian colleagues were right about one thing. Most yoga spaces are dominated by people who use them as an opportunity to *say whatever comes to mind as though that's Yoga*. And in the geographic west, where people of European descent predominate, what people in these leadership and teaching roles say are things that have *nothing to do with Yoga* and everything to do with the contingencies of their upbringing, culture, and trauma of being *W*estern. So, I could hence understand how and why my South Asian friends thought that having South Asian teachers could ameliorate this: for then, at least, whatever comes to mind and is said by these South Asian teachers will be on the basis of the South Asian tradition from where we learn about Yoga. So, it would seem that we would have a *slightly* better chance of actually learning about Yoga this way. But what these friends of mine were missing is that if the standard of teaching is just sharing *whatever comes to mind* on the basis of one's past experiences, then what we are sharing is not Yoga but our trauma responses to colonization. That is because what we acquire *passively* is not knowledge of liberation but the content of our bondage. This shows up in ordinary Yoga spaces. Here, instead of students being taught to be responsibly active, engaged participants in public life, challenging themselves while they are transparent about their own choices, which allows others to do the same, they are taught to calm the self, be in the moment, and pay attention to their emotional responses. Yoga is about being the solution of one's own life. Colonial trauma responses encourage us to be wallflowers. Most 'yoga' education is really this colonial exercise of getting us to be wallflowers.

In conversation with the Yoga scholar and ethnographer Paul Bramadat, I learned that people flock to yoga (*āsana*) studios because of an ailment or complaint, and they stay there as it appears to mitigate the pain. This leads to the confusion that the point of yoga is the reduction of suffering. In focusing on the symptom (suffering) of the injury to our personhood (a deprivation of autonomy), people who reconceive of Yoga as motivated purely for reasons of suffering reduction are like addicts with no insight into addiction: instead of looking at their own activities, choices, and priorities to make profound ethical changes so that addictive practices die a peaceful death from lack of support, their energy is focused on procuring the fix that will give them relief. And instead of solving the problem of addiction, it continues to be recharged by the delivery of the fix. Our injury to personhood is colonialism – this imposition of a perspective from the outside, which we must conform to or perish. This injury travels down to us intergenerationally, and historically as enculturation. And unless we explicate these origins, and their influence on us, we simply bring that trauma into sites of postural practice that are redefined as the paradigm case of 'yoga'. Somatization is a real psychiatric problem with real physical symptoms. Without Yoga, which helps us excavate these sources of somatic trauma, and without its practice of creating a healthy alternative that deprives our trauma of oxygen, 'yoga' practitioners perpetuate their own colonization. My hope is that with this explication of Yoga, students of Yoga will have the opportunity to do the deeper work of Yoga, which makes healing possible so that harm reduction is no longer needed.

I wish to thank some people who have supported me as I made my way into a world of interest in Yoga. First, I would like to thank Serenity Tedesco, Taina Berardi, and Prof. Christopher Key Chapple of Loyola Marymount University for choosing me as the keynote speaker for their 2020 Yoga day. I would like to thank Alyssa Wostrel for inviting me to be the keynote speaker for the 2022 Symposium on Yoga Therapy and Research (SYTAR) conference. It was there that I had the good fortune of meeting my fellow keynote speaker, Prof. Catherine Cook-Cottone, who encouraged me to write this book. I have her to thank for introducing me to her editor, Sarah Hamlin at Singing Dragon, who has been remarkably supportive in overseeing this book to publication.

I want to thank Eddie Stern, Aditi Shah, and Anusha Wijeyakumar for their friendship and support. Eddie befriended me before I became Dr Ranganathan. I taught him Philosophy and he opened the world of serious students of Yoga to me. Aditi gave me the opportunity to have smart conversations about Yoga and Philosophy on her Instagram page and that, like my experiences with Eddie, furthered my appreciation of the range of students and practitioners of Yoga. There are many smart and remarkable practitioners of Yoga out there, like Eddie and Aditi. It's one's good fortune to meet such persons. Anusha was an online supporter of my work when I was new in the online world of Yoga education, and we soon became Tamil siblings from different continents, teaching together and reflecting on the very strangeness of Yogaland. I'm grateful for her cutting insight and her low tolerance for nonsense.

I would like to thank Jeffery D. Long, Rita D. Sherma, and Christopher Jain Miller for their collegiality, friendship, and support. My York colleague and friend Prof. Alice MacLachlan deserves special recognition for encouraging me to teach diverse philosophy in 'ordinary' Philosophy courses. To Owen Ware, my University of Toronto colleague, thanks for taking the time to enter my bizarre world of being a philosopher who writes on Yoga. What's so bizarre about this, you might ask? To engage in genuine philosophical research on Yoga or any Indian philosophical tradition is to do good research and have one's work peer-reviewed by people who, more often than not, care nothing about philosophy and/or the tradition one is writing on. This is just one of the many outcomes of *W*estern colonialism.

My gurus are diverse. They are all the Philosophy professors I've ever had. I owe them my gratitude. My family too I owe gratitude for their love, support, and patience. My parents, Dr and Mrs Ranganathan, facilitated an ancestral connection to Yoga/Bhakti. For that I am grateful. My wife Andrea, my son Keshava, and my daughter Jyoti, and all of my family, have been the best well-wishers one could hope for.

I also want to express my gratitude for Yoga. While everyone else pretends being a good person, aiming for good results, and doing good things is the baseline of ethical practice, Yoga teaches us to occupy the space of failure while we do the right thing. And nothing gets better unless we have the courage to occupy that space and to do the right thing there, in failure. I wish I knew that growing up. I would have saved myself a lot of grief – the grief of holding myself to a standard of perfection that can only ever be an outcome of practice, not the condition of practice. The practice of Yoga taught me to accept failure as the place of practice. Fortunately, I learned that eventually. Unfortunately, it took decades.

I also want to thank Prof. Purushottama Bilimoria. When I was completing the manuscript for this book, he honoured me by asking me to write the foreword to his upcoming edited second volume on *Indian Ethics*. As he notes, he and I are the only two who have been at this scholarship persistently for decades. It was then important when he asked me why I chose the cover for this book that I did. Prof. Bilimoria noted that war and fighting are very small aspects of Yoga, and moreover, the Hindu Right loves to emphasize martial themes in their xenophobia. And yet, my choice of cover image, an image that brings to fore the *Mahābhārata*, the *Bhagavad Gītā*, and the war chronicled there, is martial. My response was to first note that we shouldn't let the Hindu Right and other xenophobes appropriate the tradition to the point that we are embarrassed to talk about it historically and responsibly. I explain in this book how the horse-drawn chariot with Kṛṣṇa as the charioteer is a unifying motif that calls back to the earliest articulation of Yoga in the tradition and brings to fore that Yoga is not about running away from opposition but facing challenges head on.

An animal rights activist objected to the picture as it involves horses drawing a chariot. On his view, to get horses to the point that they would participate in this endeavour is abusive. He also thought that the point of the picture was to represent my politics, when it's chosen because it is representative of the tradition. My only response to this worry about the horses is to note that our approach to nonhuman animals in a Westernized world at once denies their personhood but also imagines some natural environment in which they could do whatever they pleased without threat or coercion. Humans are imagined as the only threat entering this pristine environment and absconding with horses who would be free but for human intervention. This is, of course, not true. There is nothing safe about the natural life of any organism. In ancient South Asia and the Yoga tradition, nonhuman animals are people, just like us, and the acknowledged reality is that the world is a hostile place unless we engage in a project of solidarity with people defined by their interest in Īśvara – Sovereignty. The image shows this solidarity as an existential fact. It is not as though the interests of the horses are expendable. In this battle, Kṛṣṇa, Arjuna, and the horses share an interest in Sovereignty: they stand or fall together. Pretending that there is a safe natural environment that we can retire to is a myth that pretends that oppression isn't a reality we have to defeat. As I finish these sentences, Canada has been burning due to climate change, and climate change itself is a function of an anthropocentrism and communitarianism of the *W*estern tradition that thinks only of one's human community in an imagined otherwise pristine natural world ready for appropriation. The decolonization made possible by a real Yoga practice, that leads us to act in deference to our shared, species-transcendent interest in Sovereignty, cannot come soon enough – for the Earth, horses, and all persons.

To access the digital course in support of this book, head over to yogaphilosophy.com/courses and click on the book cover.

CHAPTER 1

INTRODUCTION: UNLEARNING COLONIALISM AND LEARNING YOGA

SYNERGIZING PRACTICE

This book is for anyone who wants a simple introduction to the philosophy of Yoga. I was motivated to write this as I found that there was no research-based, readily accessible account of Yoga and Philosophy that would be useful for teachers, practitioners, and students of Yoga, including Yoga Teacher Training programmes (YTTs). Yoga humanities and Yoga philosophy are a central part of standard teacher trainings and hence there is a need for credible material to organize lessons. Hence, this book is structured so that each chapter ends with prompts for discussion and reflection. Students and teachers can read the chapters, and teachers can lead discussions on the basis of the prompts. The chapters can be used to structure the exploration in YTTs. But any such work will also explain the basics of Yoga and Philosophy. So while my motivation for writing this is to help yoga teachers and students, anyone interested in Yoga and Philosophy will benefit from this – including students and teachers of Philosophy.

My plan in this first chapter is to introduce the topic of Yoga and Philosophy, and to then introduce this book. This overview will make the more substantial explorations in subsequent chapters easy to glide through.

As I write this, there is a deficit of credible material for learning about Yoga and Philosophy. The vast majority of authors, even in Yoga Studies, who claim to have something to say about Yoga and Philosophy, are not scholars of Philosophy, and hence they cannot be scholars of Yoga, the philosophy. And yet, there are volumes written on the topic. Why there is a deficit in credible, research-based knowledge about Yoga and Philosophy is something that we must address as students of Yoga. The short answer is: colonialism. Philosophy like any academic subject takes years of research, and to become an expert in it one must become a philosopher, writing, engaging in, and producing philosophical research as a contribution to scholarship. But colonialism doesn't like Philosophy because Philosophy raises awkward questions that colonialism can't handle. In a colonized world, a purely philosophical approach to anything is discouraged. While students of Philosophy are widely known to be top of the list in a variety of standardized tests and competencies,[1] colonialism tries to describe Philosophy as a waste of time. And yet, philosophical skills enable Philosophy students to reinvent themselves, problem solve, and create opportunities for themselves. Hence, they typically move on to many successful pursuits. It's just not the case that these are labelled 'philosophy' so it's hard to track all these successful philosophers in public life. One of my goals in this book is to help yoga practitioners tap into the benefits that Philosophy facilitates, and this has much to do with the teachings of Yoga, a particular philosophy from ancient South Asia. As we shall see, following the teachings of Yoga is necessary to be a competent philosopher. A competent philosopher understands all sorts of options and gets over their own ego as a barrier to understanding.

Yoga, the philosophy, is an ancient option from the South Asian tradition, and quite unique to it. Classical sources for this philosophy include the Vedas (especially the *Upaniṣads*) (1500–500 BCE), written in Vedic, epics such as the *Mahābhārata*, which contains within it the famous *Bhagavad Gītā* (300 BCE–300 CE), and the systematic and formal account by Patañjali in the *Yoga Sūtra* (200 BCE–200 CE), written in Sanskrit. What is often called 'yoga' these days consists of the descendant practices of the philosophy, Yoga. Most people come to Yoga via postural practices (*āsana*), or breathing exercises (*prāṇāyāma*), or perhaps mental practices of mind focus (*saṃyamaḥ*) often called meditation. Fun fact: the ancient South Asian (Vedic and Sanskrit) word for meditation is 'yoga'. So when you are practising yoga, you are engaging in a meditative exercise. But importantly, these various exercises that people label as 'yoga' are *ways to practise* an ancient philosophy, Yoga. This means that the usual way of framing the topic of yoga as primarily a postural, breathing, or mental exercise gets things backwards. It is easy to misunderstand the point. The problem is not in thinking that postural exercises, breathing exercises, or the training of the mind are ways to practise Yoga. They are. The inaccuracy consists in thinking that those exercises are the paradigm cases of yoga, and that the philosophy of Yoga is an inessential enrichment. The problem with this way of thinking of yoga is that it renders unclear why anything could ever count as a practice of yoga in the first place. Everyone sits and most people move; that doesn't mean they are practising *āsana* (postural exercises). Everyone alive breathes; it doesn't follow that everyone is practising *prāṇāyāma* (breathing exercises). We all take time to focus our mind on things of interest; that doesn't mean we're engaging in meditation. Something turns ordinary activities that people can do into the practice of yoga. That is the philosophy, capital 'Y' Yoga. When we practise the philosophy, Yoga, we live our life within this philosophy. Then activities we do turn into ways to practise Yoga, and we might call these activities small 'y' yoga, such as *āsana* and *prāṇāyāma*. Thus, if one wishes to learn yoga and teach yoga, one must understand the philosophy, Yoga, as the basis of the practice.

- The analysis presented here will be short and easy to understand.

It will be easy to understand, as it will lay out in simple language the basics of Yoga the philosophy and practice, and the contrary options that one needs to understand as distinct from Yoga.

- But it will be challenging and force you to think, because understanding the philosophy of Yoga involves unlearning colonialism.

In some cases, this exploration of Yoga and Philosophy will constitute a significant heightening of the bar of what counts as the baseline of understanding Yoga. Since teaching Yoga and Philosophy publicly, I have found that average yoga students, teachers, and practitioners are completely up for the challenge. But it will be a challenge.

For those who are accustomed to participating in colonialism (and we all do this to varying degrees), the difference between what we learn from Yoga, the original decolonial philosophy, and the beliefs we have as a result of colonization will produce a weird experience. This does not mean that you are misunderstanding what you are reading. Quite the opposite. You are rather contending with the incongruity of your beliefs with what you are learning. For those of us who love Philosophy – and Yoga – that's a welcome discomfort of *tapas* (Sanskrit for 'heat production' – going against the grain, being unconservative). We engage in *tapas* when we lean into a challenging posture or get a good workout at the gym – and when we are being philosophical!

Yoga is about being an independent individual (this is called *kaivalya* in Sanskrit). Colonialism is the opposing project of one power imposing its views on how to live on a population so they are no longer independent.[2] When it is successful, the colonizing project, its values, and its outlook are localized by the colonized as their values and outlook. The project is violent and involves erasing various aspects of people's rich lives to make way for colonization. *W*estern colonialism is the project of imposing a *W*estern outlook on everything. Most people speak simply about the west and by that they mean Europe and its political and ethnic descendants. But the geography of the west contains more than people of European dissent. It contains Africa and Indigenous peoples of North and South America. In other words, Black, Indigenous, and People of Colour (BIPOC) are originally western too and *W*estern colonialism tries to hide that. Hence, I recommend distinguishing the mere geography of the west with a colonizing tradition with roots in ancient Greek thought: the *W*est. This is the capital '*W*' that leans on the 'est'. In a world dominated by the *W*est, it is easy to simply participate in this tradition by passively taking on its perspective, as encouraged by our upbringings that have themselves been impacted by *W*estern colonialism. Then one tries to understand Yoga not in terms of what it has to teach us but in terms of beliefs that we gain from our *W*esternized traditions. As the *W*est has been a global colonizing force for millennia, and has a long history of colonizing South Asia, from where Yoga comes, nowhere is immune from its influence and students of Yoga must be especially mindful of its interference. Without the original practice of Yoga, that teaches us how to be aware of and protect our individuality from external influences, we end up participating in *W*estern colonialism by passively endorsing and using its beliefs in our project of understanding. Protecting our own independence is a choice but one we have to affirm to learn anything, including Yoga. Otherwise, all we are doing is reapplying second-hand beliefs from colonization we gain passively.

In the next section, we will move on to a synopsis of Yoga and its opposite: colonialism. We will conclude this chapter with the contrast between Philosophy and colonialism.

YOGA: THE ORIGINAL DECOLONIAL PRACTICE

The *Yoga Sūtra* begins by presenting us with a choice. We can either delineate and identify various practical and philosophical options that we can choose from, thereby protecting our freedom of choice, or we can passively identify with our experiences as though they inform us of our options. Unless we make the effort to delineate and organize the options, we are passively influenced by our experiences as though they teach us something about ourselves. When we organize the data to appreciate the options, our experiences do not teach us: our organizational activity teaches us. Deferring to our experiences, rather than our activity, is to accept a passive approach to life. This is to simply identify with whatever we observe and feel. Yoga (the *metaethics* or practice of understanding the practical options) is the practice of delineating options to protect personal freedom. It is the life of organized and integrative activity. Anti-yoga is about giving up this freedom by being influenced by our experiences (YS I.2–4).

Why is being influenced by our experiences not good for us? The problem with our experiences is that they are not completely up to us as they are often the result of many factors, including other people's choices. To identify with such experiences is to passively take on external factors (called nature, or *prakṛti* in Yoga) and other people's choices as though they are part of our own self-understanding. According to Yoga, this basic ignorance (*avidyā*) of anti-Yoga leads to a false sense of self called *egotism* (*asmitā* in Sanskrit). Importantly, egotism involves the *internalization* of external experiences. On the basis of egotism, we are relieved by what is in conformity with our experience-internalized-sense-of-self and alarmed by what is not in conformity to it. As colonialism is the imposition of a perspective on the colonized, identifying with our experiences – anti-Yoga – and the subsequent formation of an ego is the mechanism by which colonialism succeeds. In this case, we internalize the external colonial order.

Western colonialism has impacted every continent of the globe. Hence, the experiences one has on every continent are likely to be structured by Western colonialism. When we identify with our experiences structured by Western colonialism, we internalize Western colonialism as part of our ego. We find ourselves relieved when the world conforms to these colonial expectations and alarmed when it does not. But either way, we are stuck in a state of affliction (*kleśa* in Sanskrit), which we call trauma (YS II.3). As this trauma is a function of identifying with the regularities of colonialism, we should call this particular kind of trauma *colonial trauma.* But even apart from any explicit experience of colonialism, egotism is a colonized self – a self colonized by the experiences of the world. Anti-yoga is ordinary. It is how we live when we do not make the effort to practise Yoga. And hence, it's very ordinary for people coming to Yoga to bring their colonial trauma with them as they try to study Yoga. But even otherwise, in failing to practise Yoga, we simply identify with and participate in the systemic oppression of our world as we use it to inform our sense of self. Instead of identifying with our interests as independent people, with anti-Yoga we identify with the space left to us by oppression.

Racialized people, or people from marginalized groups, are continuously told by others to occupy a smaller space left to them by a world of discrimination. If they end up identifying with those experiences, they will think that what the external world teaches them (about their inferiority) is true about who they are. Then, they will *ironically* act in ways that support and affirm that marginalized understanding. They will feel ironically happy when their subordination and marginalization is affirmed and alarmed if they have to confront and challenge it, to the point that they will put energy into resisting being political and standing up for themselves. They will lash out at the very thought that they have to change. According to Yoga, this is a result of the formation of an ego on the basis of oppressive experiences. However, Yoga teaches us that people in positions of privilege have the same problem to deal with. Their egotism may in some ways be harder to overcome because their experiences are supportive of their ego.

As an example of this, consider the wonderful analysis by the philosopher Grant Silva in his paper titled 'Racism as Self-Love' (2019).[3] Silva points out that we ordinarily think of racism as a kind of hatred of people of a certain race. But this overlooks the ways in which individuals can be racist out of a concern for their self based on a false self-understanding. Specifically, Silva focuses on people being racist not because they hate Black people but because (they believe) they love themselves as a White person. Silva's example is amenable to a Yoga analysis. In this case, a racist White person who doesn't hate Black people identifies with their own representation as a 'White' person within a world structured by White Supremacy, which is a political order created by Western colonialism. Once a White individual identifies with their experience within a world of White Supremacy as top of the heap, they internalize this political structure as their egotism. But then, they are happy when things conform to their racist expectations and alarmed when, for instance, they perceive Black people on equal footing, and hence feel the need to cross the street to avoid being close to them. Something like this happens to very many students of Yoga who identify with the West. Here, they are happy when what they learn reinforces Western supremacy and alarmed when they have to learn about South Asian philosophy, such as Yoga. On the Yoga analysis, this happens because of an internalization of an external colonial order. When we become colonized, we act as though our self-interest is the same as the external political order.

The *Yoga Sūtra*, the systematic account of the philosophy of Yoga, teaches us that anti-Yoga can be avoided, and we can practise the metaethics of Yoga by committing to the (ideal) normative ethics of Yoga. A normative ethical theory tells us what to do and what to aim for. An ideal normative ethical theory specifies what to do and aim for in ideal circumstances. Yoga as an ideal normative theory tells us that when we are practising Yoga, we are primarily devoted to the ideal of Sovereignty or Lordliness, Īśvara (in Sanskrit). Īśvara is the ideal of what it is to be a functional person. It is characterized by two sets of traits: on the one hand, it is not constrained by its past, and hence it's free to move forward. On the other hand, its activities are not afflicted but rather a matter of self-governance. Hence, in practising devotion to Īśvara (*Īśvara praṇidhāna*), we also practise its two essential traits of unconservatism (*tapas*) and self-governance (*svādhyāya*) (YS II.1). As we practise self-governance, we acknowledge and own the values that we set ourselves (YS II.44).

Īśvara is not the same as our ego created by our contingent experiences, but is the practical interest that all people share. Therefore, devotion to Īśvara is a state of *solidarity* with all persons. Importantly, perfecting this practice is a matter of an ethical cleansing that leads us away from all selfishness in every context (called the *dharmameghasamādhi* in Sanskrit). The outcome of this practice is our own autonomy or independence – *kaivalya* in Sanskrit (YS IV.29–34).

What is so important about learning about the actual philosophy of Yoga is that it teaches us that *anything* and *everything* we need to do to live our lives is an opportunity to practise Yoga. Everything we do, whether spending time with friends or family, getting an education, pursuing hobbies, earning a living, is an opportunity for us to practise Yoga. For anything we must do for ourselves we can do as part of our devotion to Īśvara, while practising its essential traits of unconservatism and self-governance. Of course, some things might be incompatible with this practice – and that's what we need to change in our lives. That is why Yoga is the original decolonial practice. It allows everything except for our internalization of oppression, which is the opposite of devotion to Īśvara. But everything else can be a small 'y' practice of yoga for us. Importantly, Yoga teaches us that self-care and concern for other people are not mutually exclusive. Rather, in understanding oneself as a person with an interest in Īśvara, we come to perceive what we have in common with others: an interest in Sovereignty. In other words, Yoga teaches us that the more committed we are to ourselves as an individual person – the more we value ourselves – the more connected with and concerned for others we are too.

A person, Yoga teaches us, is defined as something that thrives given their own Īśvara, given their own unconservatism and self-governance. Unlike plants that thrive when they are stuck in the ground they were planted in and given valuable environments, persons are the kinds of things that thrive when they are not stuck in their past and are free to determine their own choices and values. Yoga leads us to appreciate that persons come in all genders, sexes, skin colours, *and species*. The Earth, for instance, is a person on the Yoga account, as are most nonhuman animals. South Asians in general did not think that there was anything particularly special about being human. For the prioritization of humans, anthropocentrism, we have to look to the West (as we shall see in the next chapter). But this radically simple idea of personhood forms the basis of a lot of what people think of as progressive philosophy and politics today. But it does not stop there. What people think of as essential to social justice also comes down to us from the *Yoga Sūtra*.

In addition to an ideal normative ethical theory, Patañjali, the author of the *Yoga Sūtra*, sets out what we today in Philosophy call a nonideal ethical theory: an ethical theory that we have to make use of in imperfect times. Patañjali describes this as a remedy (*upāya*) to use to help with failing practice. This is what he calls the *Eight Limbs of Yoga* (*aṣṭāṅga yoga*). The first limb, called *Yama*, he prescribes as a universal obligation. Accordingly, we ought to first begin by disrupting systemic harm (*ahiṃsā*) to allow us to participate in the moral facts (*satya*) that do not deprive others of their requirements (*asteya*), and respect personal boundaries that allow for learning (*brahmacarya*) that leads us away from appropriation (*aparigrahā*). Further, Patañjali notes that when people are opposed to disrupting systemic harm by promoting violence, they do so on the basis of past trauma. The Yogi recognizes this root of violence in past trauma and then sets themselves out to be an opponent to such trauma and violence by living in a contrary manner. This has the effect of getting the opponent to renounce their hostility (YS II.30–35). If this sounds familiar to you, that is because M. K. Gandhi based his political philosophy on the *Yoga Sūtra* and the teachings of Patañjali. His *Collected Works* are filled with references to Patañjali and the *Yoga Sūtra* as the origins of his thinking on political matters. On this basis, he organized the mass project of Indian civil disobedience aimed at getting the British to quit their colonial hold on South Asia. It worked. But importantly too, Gandhi's struggle (which he called *satyagraha*, or the way of truth) was an inspiration to M. L. King, the famous American Civil Rights leader, who modelled his political struggle to end segregation and other legal forms of racial discrimination in the US – also an example of Western colonialism – on Gandhi's project.[4] Nowadays it is common for progressive activists to take these political struggles rooted in *ahiṃsā*, or the disruption of systemic harm, as their model, and to use the disruption of systemic harm as their political programme. The world over, these projects can be traced back to the *Yoga Sūtra* and the classical philosophy of Yoga.

So not only do we learn from Yoga that it is wrong to discriminate against people on the basis of appearance, for a person is not how they look but what accounts for their thriving (Īśvara), we also learn about the political means to address the systemic harm of colonialism by practising the disruption of systemic harm. We learn from Yoga that our interests in being quirky individuals is something we share with all individuals.

After the first limb, Patañjali prescribes a second limb that involves an uncompromising (*śauca*) and contented (*santoṣa*) commitment to the core normative theory of Yoga: Devotion to Sovereignty (*Īśvara praṇidhāna*) and the practice of unconservatism (*tapas*) and self-governance (*svādhyāya*). The third limb is *Āsana*, which is described as taking up the space of one's life made possible by the previous limbs (YS II.32–44). Today, '*āsana*' is the term used to cover postural exercise.

Learning *āsana* as a postural practice is a small way that we can make room for ourselves as practitioners of Yoga. There are many others, and any of them are ways to practise Yoga as a Devotion to Sovereignty. After learning about the ways in which Yoga in the first instance is this ancient philosophy from South Asia, and derivatively postural exercises, I find some people get confused. They wonder: can I continue to teach and practise *āsana* as though it is yoga? Certainly. Before teaching *āsana* or practising it, engage in this framing exercise by saying and affirming:

> *Yoga is the ancient philosophy that teaches us that all right choosing and doing occurs within the context of devotion to Īśvara (Sovereignty, Lordliness, Independence), and as part of this practice, we also set ourselves to practise its essential traits of tapas (unconservatism) and svādhyāya (self-governance). Now we will practise* _____ (fill in the blank with your practice, such as postures, breathing exercises, mind-focusing routines) *as a way to explore this devotional practice.*

See? So easy. The idea that there is some profound incongruity between practising yoga and understanding the philosophy of Yoga is not true. But what is certain is that without understanding the philosophy of Yoga, we won't understand how practising yoga is a way to explore our own independence. If we do not understand this, we might be repeating something like *āsana* while participating in our own colonization.

LEARNING YOGA AND PHILOSOPHY

Philosophy consists in using logic, which concerns how we *ought to think*, to sort out topics that are controversial. Such topics include metaphysics (which asks what is reality), epistemology (which asks what is knowledge), and ethics, which investigates the Right thing to choose and do, and the Good thing to aim for and value. Philosophy is not primarily descriptive. It rather helps us understand logical implications of assumptions that, if we're not conscious of them, structure our lives. Yoga the philosophy makes clear what is involved in engaging in the discipline of Philosophy, as it helps us render explicit assumptions, which we can then contemplate.

Perhaps the most toxic function of Western colonization is that it ends up labelling itself, the Western tradition, as a universal, secular, standard of humanity and 'Philosophy', whereas anything from outside of the West is labelled as religion or spirituality. BIPOC traditions are then not understood in terms of their contributions to Philosophy but by way of their deviation from or conformity to the Western tradition. This effectively blocks BIPOC traditions from offering moral and political criticisms of Western colonialism, as they are marginalized as irrelevant to secular life.[5] As Yoga is an ancient South Asian philosophy, it too is treated as a marginal activity, that is spiritual or religious, and not as central to ordinary life. This sets up the discriminatory expectation that the study of Yoga and other BIPOC traditions has to occur *outside of and without Philosophy*, and within inter-disciplines such as Religious Studies, Indology, or Yoga Studies. As most folks do not practise Yoga but rather identify with their beliefs facilitated by their experiences – which for almost everyone today is a function of Western colonialism – most defend this subterfuge as part of their egotism. This means that they are happy when the West is treated as a universal standard of humanity and upset when it isn't. As Western colonialism is a global phenomenon, this reaction is common throughout the world. One nontrivial outcome of this phenomenon is that Yoga is *re-presented* in terms of its conformity to and deviation from the Western tradition. It usually comes as news to most that what is familiarly marketed as yoga is really some version of Plato or Aristotle. This is its supposed conformity to the West. It is also represented as religious or spiritual. This is its deviation. Both obfuscate actual Yoga. The way to fight this subterfuge is to learn Philosophy. Philosophy is decolonial, and Yoga, the philosophy, helps us understand what the disciplinary activity of Philosophy is. As we practise Yoga, we practise being philosophers.

'Philosophy' is a Greek word that means 'love of wisdom'. It has two different uses. According to the common use, 'philosophy' is a perspective. One could have a philosophy about home decoration or gardening according to this usage. The basic meaning of 'Philosophy' is that it is a discipline in which we can critically inspect theories about topics that are definable in terms of their disagreements. When we are philosophical in the disciplinary sense, we can and should learn about many contrasting theories and we can maintain our own independence from what we are considering. Just as biologists are specialists in the discipline of Biology, mathematicians are specialists in the discipline of Mathematics, philosophers are specialists in the discipline of Philosophy. And to become such a specialist, one has to contribute to the respective field of research by engaging in the discipline. So biologists earn their PhD in Biology by contributing to the field of Biology. Philosophers similarly have to make such a contribution themselves to Philosophy to become experts. My PhD dissertation in Philosophy was on the topic of translating philosophy, and the contribution I made was by formulating and defending a general theory of understanding and reproducing texts from languages and cultures that we share nothing with. No one had done this work before. The project required understanding of thoughts, arguments, and art from other times and cultures without the narcissism of projecting our beliefs on to them. This research was essential in facilitating my knowledge of Yoga in the original Sanskrit texts.

The obstacle to understanding how we can learn from the ancient texts of Yoga philosophy is an ancient theory of thought in the Western tradition, which identifies thought with speech. This Linguistic Account of Thought (LAT) is captured in the ancient Greek idea of *logos* (one word for thought, reason, and speech). Accordingly, thought is what we are inclined to say.[6] Thoughts, such as *it is raining outside* have two important properties. First, they can be true or false. Second, they can logically entail other thoughts. So, whether or not it is true, if it is true that *it is raining outside*, we can infer that *water is falling from the sky*. The former thought provides inferential support for the latter. We can contrast thoughts such as these with a belief, which is the attitude of endorsing a thought. If *I believe it is raining outside*, I take the thought to be true. A belief however is an attitude toward thoughts (what are called propositional attitudes). And there are many, such as *hope* and *fear*. Unlike thoughts, nothing follows from a propositional attitude. If *I believe it is raining outside*, it doesn't follow that *water is falling from the sky*. My belief is really about my attitude and psychology of what is true, not about the rain, and not what we can reason about.

To make this clear, consider two different *deductive* arguments:

Premise 1: The Moon is a squash.
Premise 2: Squashes grow on trees.
Conclusion: The Moon grows on a tree.

Everything said here is false. However, if the two premises are true, we can infer the conclusion. This argument is *logically valid*. A valid logical argument is an argument where *if* the premises are true, the conclusion has to be true. Valid arguments can be comprised of entirely false propositions, like this one. Now consider an argument where everything is true:

Premise 1: Biden was POTUS in 2021.
Premise 2: Modi was PM of India in 2021.
Conclusion: Shyam Ranganathan is the author of this book.

While everything said here is true, the argument is invalid: even if the premises are true, the conclusion does not have to be true. In other words, it's true but nonsense. Logically invalid arguments can be comprised of entirely true propositions, like this one. This shows that saying or believing true things is not the same as being reasonable. We call this error of thinking that truth is primary in reasoning the *truth fallacy*. When we engage in the truth fallacy, we simply confuse what is true about our world (or at least, how we see it) with what is reasonable.

To be clear, and we will review this later, there are many forms of reasoning (including induction and abduction). Deduction, of which validity is its standard, is just one. However, what distinguishes all forms of reason from irrationality is that reason is about *inferential support*. Thoughts (reasons) can provide inferential support for other thoughts even if they are false. And many true claims can fail to provide other true claims with inferential support.

- Reason (inferential support) and truth are two separate criteria for the evaluation of thoughts, and when we engage in the truth fallacy, we treat the criterion of whether a thought is true or not as a criterion to evaluate its reasonableness, which is a mistake.

This is one of the first things Philosophy professors try to teach their students in logic, in critical thinking classes, and in introduction to Philosophy. It's a tough lesson to learn as, culturally, especially in the West, there is a strong predilection to engage in the truth fallacy. Worse, in academia, where authors really should know better, it is common for authors writing on Yoga and South Asian philosophy to engage in this fallacy. I've made a career writing about this.

The idea that good explanations are explanations in terms of what we believe is called *interpretation*. It is widely acclaimed in recent Western philosophy, even though it demonstrably violates exactly what philosophers teach in logic classes.[7] What we ought to engage in, in contrast, is *explication*, which is to use our logical skills to render explicit ideas, theories, and options. This is core to Philosophy. It is also just plain reasonable. It is also what we are doing now. We are using logical skills to distinguish between models of explanation (such as interpretation) and models of thought (such as LAT) to understand their limitations and their practical implications. And in so delineating these options, we don't have to buy them. In effect, by explicating, we are engaging in Yoga as the responsible activity of organizing our experiences (which includes these theories such as LAT and interpretation) to make room for ourselves. But instead, what we find in the Western tradition is the predominance of interpretation and a minimization of the importance of Philosophy. In contrast to South Asia, where philosophers were revered, from the very start of the *W*estern tradition, beginning with Socrates, there was an intolerance to free thinking, as evidenced in a succession of public executions of intellectuals (Socrates, Jesus, Boethius, Hypatia...). In effect, to be part of the *W*estern tradition is to buy its beliefs, and those who do not are treated as a threat to this tradition. And this model of understanding, interpretation, is the kernel of anti-Yoga. When we explicate, we do not identify with our experiences but rather organize thinking. When we interpret, we are literally influenced by our beliefs.

Why is there such a strong connection between interpretation (the truth fallacy) and the *W*estern tradition? It has to do with LAT, which is at the heart of the *W*estern tradition. When we want to say that 'It is true that it is raining outside', we just say 'It is raining outside.' The pragmatic force of saying 'It is raining outside' is to articulate our belief that it is true that it is raining outside. LAT, which conflates thought with speech, removes a clear distinction between the thought *it is raining outside* and my *belief that it is raining outside*. Once the thought and its belief are not clearly distinguished, then every explanation by way of thought is an explanation by way of belief: which is interpretation. Put another way, what LAT does is it leads us to believe that a good explanation of everything is framed in terms of what *I would say*. As this model of thought is steeped in the *W*estern tradition, as the *W*estern tradition spreads it does so by explaining everything in terms of what *it would say*, which is what it takes to be true. As colonialism is the imposition of a perspective on others, as the *W*estern tradition spreads by LAT and the interpretations it generates, it imposes its beliefs on everything else. This not only renders it difficult to understand others who do not share our beliefs, it also forces us and them to conform to those beliefs.

- And so we see that the *W*estern tradition becomes a global colonizing tradition because of a seemingly innocent model of thought (LAT) that leads to interpretation.
- Aside from being the core of anti-Yoga, and an origin of irrationality, interpretation is the kernel of colonialism.

So the first order of business is to understand the roots of the *W*estern tradition in our next chapter, '*W*estern *Saṃskāra*-s – *W*estern Colonialism'. *Saṃskāra* is a rite, or a practice, but in the *Yoga Sūtra*, it stands for interpretation

– a knee-jerk, subconscious explanation of experiences in terms of beliefs and other attitudes toward thoughts. We might decide to install habits, or *saṃskāra*-s, as an antidote to *saṃskāra*-s that are formed passively. In this case, we are in charge. But a life based on *saṃskāra,* especially when we are not in control, is problematic as it recreates our expectation by only allowing what is consistent with our expectations. As interpretation, it is also irrational as it engages the *truth fallacy.*

What distinguishes my research, teaching, and publications is that I make the *saṃskāra*-s that interfere with credible research my focus, and in a Westernized world our *saṃskāra*-s are Western. Given its roots in LAT, Western scholarship on Yoga switches focus from Philosophy to Linguistic topics, such as Sanskrit, and Philology, while employing interpretation. The result is a literature on Yoga that is uninterested in Philosophy and proceeds by interpreting from a Western vantage – all the while cloaking this by an ostensible concern for South Asian languages and culture (itself a focus generated by LAT).[8] Without calling out and explicitly identifying the *saṃskāra*-s we employ, we'll simply reapply them and then there's no learning: only colonization. As our *saṃskāra*-s in a Westernized world are Western, we need to begin by studying these. Hence, we shall revisit LAT and appreciate its role in the formation of the philosophies of Plato (who modelled education as a pyramid scheme with an enlightened guru at the top, who sets out a curriculum that participants are challenged to master in order to climb the organization's rungs) and Aristotle (who conceived of learning as a matter of having the right cultural experiences). LAT problematizes outsiders who do not share our language and hence who literally cannot say what we say. Both Plato's and Aristotle's views problematize the outsider. The Romans who began unpacking the colonialism of the Western tradition arrived at a solution for accommodating outsider traditions that they colonized. The ones that were tolerated (though not all were) as subservient were recognized as having *religio* – tradition. It's from the Roman Empire that we get our idea of religion. People talk about religion as though it is something all traditions and societies have, but it is just the way the West subordinated outsiders it didn't exterminate.[9]

As I point out in my book, *Hinduism: A Contemporary Philosophical Investigation* (2018), as the West spreads while continuing the project of the Roman Empire, it brands all BIPOC traditions as 'religious' or spiritual, and it treats itself as the default, universal, or secular tradition. As evidence, you could draw up a list of world religions: Judaism, Christianity, Islam, Zoroastrianism,

Buddhism, Jainism, Hinduism, Taoism, Shintoism, Confucianism... *all BIPOC*, all originally non-*W*estern. And I show that the same positions (atheist or Theist) are called secular or religious depending upon whether they are *W*estern or BIPOC. Call this Secularism$_2$: this is the idea that something is religious if it is not *W*estern, which effectively includes all BIPOC traditions, while the secular is conflated with the *W*estern tradition. Religions so dubbed are not explicated and understood as contributing to philosophical options. They are rather interpreted either as conforming to or deviating from the *W*est. The more they deviate, the more religious and spiritual they are said to be. The more culturally alien they are, the more they deviate. In contrast, ancient South Asians got along with each other by explicating, and they had a tradition we could call Secularism$_1$: free and open philosophical exploration. South Asians had no official position they shared: they took contrasting views on various philosophical matters. But continuing with the project of *W*estern colonialism, the British decided to follow the Roman example and classify South Asia as a religion. So they used a Persian word, 'Hindu', which roughly means 'India', to name being Indian as a religion. Defining people in terms of their geography is a key part of racial identity.[10] Racial identities, unlike ethnic identities, come from the outside, and people have little agency over this.[11] There is hence something importantly racial about this categorization of South Asia as Hindu. But as it comes to South Asians via colonialism, it becomes part of South Asian colonial trauma – something we need to be aware of when we try to track what is happening in South Asia today with the rise of the Hindu Right (which we shall address). By this colonial minting of 'Hinduism', Yoga and all Indigenous South Asian positions are Hindu. So too, by extension, is the ten-numeral place system where numbers are represented by a combination of 0, 1, 2, 3, 4, 5, 6, 7, 8, and 9.

The reason this is all important is that in a *W*esternized world, *W*esternized students of yoga seek out gurus who run pyramid schemes where learning yoga is about understanding how to fit into the organization, or they seek out exotic cultural experiences (usually South Asian) that they imitate by changing their dress, names, or greetings (to 'namaste') as though that's learning Yoga. That's just Plato and Aristotle, not Yoga. But these *W*estern models of yoga education are also the sites of abuse, and scandals, because these models have no way to distinguish between the authority of such organizations to enforce opinions and expertise in Yoga. Once a student is in the pyramid scheme, 'learning' about yoga is just about social conformity to organizational expectations – the very opposite of Yoga! This conflation of knowledge, or critical thinking, with belief is an outcome of LAT. Similarly, yoga students, given the *West*'s rebranding of South Asia as a religion, Hinduism, are understandably confused about whether Yoga is religious and spiritual or secular. And in a Secular$_2$ world where the secular is the *Western*, Yoga seems like a threat to secularism and is hence barred from being taught in schools in some jurisdictions. But this is a bit of colonial nonsense that is not easy to criticize unless we understand the *Western* *saṃskāra*-s at work. Without acknowledging this, we are left with an impossible choice of affirming either that yoga is religious (Hindu) or that it is secular, but not both. Explicated, we will see how both are true, just as numbers are both secular and Hindu. Hence, both yoga and numbers can and should be taught to children in secular education!

By identifying how much of 'yoga education' and the usual pretence of doing yoga ('namaste') is really just the *West* and its *saṃskāra*-s, we can then see that the usual depiction of Yoga as an exercise in mysticism or spirituality is a colonial ruse. Yoga is about developing our critical thinking skills so that we can be effective individuals. And this transformation is entirely ethical (a *dharmameghasamādhi* in Sanskrit, YS IV.29), but the ethics of this process are not defined by familiar ethical theories in the *West*. As we practise Yoga, we uncover our interpretations that hinder understanding and thereby free ourselves of those defects. This is decolonial. If we do not do this, we live by these interpretations. If we explicate the *Yoga Sūtra*, we can see this is how Yoga is defined at the very start (YS I.2–4). So it is fitting that we revisit the explication and interpretation distinction as modern ways to talk about Yoga and anti-Yoga. That will be the first order of business in Chapter 3, 'Yoga as a Basic Ethical (Dharma) Theory'. With the help of wonderful scholars, I used explication to structure an important contribution to research that I edited: *The Bloomsbury Research Handbook of Indian Ethics* (2017). When I began my education, the dominant view in the literature was that South Asians were religious and had no interest in ethical questions. What we find, when we explicate, is that in addition to three familiar ethical theories of Virtue Ethics (the good agent is the condition of right choice), Consequentialism (the right thing to do is justified by the good), and Deontology (while there are many good things to do or allow, only some are right, and these are our duties or rights), there is a fourth theory that is unique to the South Asian tradition. This is Yoga (also called Bhakti or devotion), sourced from the

Vedas, *Upaniṣads*, *Yoga Sūtra*, and *Bhagavad Gītā*. Here we will review contrary South Asian options, such as Buddhism and Jainism, and appreciate the ways in which these are distinct ethical theories from Yoga. Of special interest are Sāṅkhya and Vedānta, which are often conflated with Yoga but are importantly distinct. Yoga affirms the importance of agency and practice: Sāṅkhya denies it. Interpreted, all of these positions are represented as a singular, vague, spiritual, obtuse mishmash doled out to students of yoga who are thereby confused.

In Chapter 4, '*Yoga Sūtra*: Activism and Social Justice (Books 1 and 2)', we can take a closer look at the first two of the four books of the *Yoga Sūtra*. Here, students will be provided with an overview of the main ideas explicated in the *Yoga Sūtra* that have to do with the moral and political aspects of Yoga. We will cover the first five of the Eight Limbs of Yoga: *Yama*, *Niyama*, *Āsana*, *Prāṇāyāma*, and *Pratyāhāra*. (When I am referring to any of these Limbs, such as *Āsana* or *Prāṇāyāma* as standalone practices separated from Yoga, I will decapitalize, and talk of *āsana* or *prāṇāyāma*.)

A theme that emerges throughout the *Yoga Sūtra* is that the opposite of the ethical life of Yoga is violence and trauma. It has become popular to speak about a special kind of Yoga instruction that is informed by trauma, as though there's some type of Yoga that is ignorant of trauma. It is rather more appropriate to inform our trauma with our Yoga, as it's the Yoga that dispels the ignorance of trauma. Part of what sustains the idea that Yoga has to be informed by trauma is the conflation of Yoga with ableism – the idea that there are some types of abilities that are assumed, basic, and essential to being a person, while yoga is an exercise of those abilities. Yoga, in contrast, is anti-ableist. It identifies people not with abilities but with their interest in Īśvara. Understanding the primacy of Yoga to diagnosing and curing trauma is of first importance to yoga therapy but also teachers of yoga who are *always* faced with a class of students with some degree of trauma. Our exploration of the *Yoga Sūtra* will help facilitate an understanding of the ways in which trauma – *kleśa* to use the yoga term – is often normalized as part of the legacy of colonialism.

In Chapter 5, '*Yoga Sūtra*: Self-Care (Books 3 and 4)', we move to the last two books of the *Yoga Sūtra*, where the theme is about how the practice of Yoga supports the practitioner to live a full and complete personal life, which includes material success. We will focus on the text and observe that by the end of the Yoga process, final independence (*kaivalya*) is brought about by an ethical transformation (*dharmameghasamādhi*) (YS IV.29–34). Here, the remaining three of the Eight Limbs of Yoga of *Dhāraṇā*, *Dhyāna*, and *Samādhi* are reviewed.

Students will learn about the extended commentarial tradition starting with Vyāsa and how in Western, colonial discourse on Yoga, these commentaries that often deny the importance of agency and activism are mixed up with the moral transformative emphasis of Yoga.

No account of Yoga philosophy would be complete without examining the argument in the *Bhagavad Gītā* (300 BCE–300 CE) for Yoga (called *Bhakti Yoga* in this text). But to understand this important contribution, we have to understand that it's just a chapter in a wider epic, the *Mahābhārata*, and the entire epic is a thought experiment about the problems of conventional morality focused on good character (Virtue Ethics), good outcomes (Consequentialism), and good rules (Deontology). In a Westernized world, conventional morality dominates. But the Yoga tradition teaches us that people worried about being conventionally good are easy targets for manipulation by moral parasites, who want others to be good so they can be taken advantage of. This creates a context of violence and oppression. The *Bhagavad Gītā*, a dialogue between Kṛṣṇa (who embodies *tapas* and Īśvara) and his student Arjuna, teaches us that sometimes we have to take a stand against oppression when everything starts to fall apart, and what helps us put things back together is Yoga. Specifically, as the title of Chapter 6 says, sometimes we have to 'Take the Fight to the Problem: *Bhagavad Gītā* and Yoga'. As we explore this material, we will also learn how the seeds of these insights and arguments were already sown in the dialectic and change in the Vedas and *Upaniṣads*.

In Chapter 7, '"Modern Yoga" and Colonial Trauma', we shall consider the history of what gets called 'modern yoga' or 'modern postural yoga' in Western colonialism. In the last chapter, Chapter 8, 'Being an Authentic Yoga Teacher, Student, and Practitioner', we bring the threads of our various investigations together and address the question of what it is to be a teacher, student, and practitioner of yoga.

CHAPTER 1 REFLECTIONS

- What were your first impressions of yoga? Did you think that yoga was something everyone should do, or only those who prefer it?
- What characterized your entry into this topic? Did you learn 'yoga' first

and then Yoga? If you learned it this way, how different would that be from learning about Yoga first and then various forms of yoga?

» What were your first impressions of Philosophy? Did you think it was about your beliefs and how you see things?

» Here is a claim we will be investigating: *Being reasonable (logical) and practising Yoga, the philosophy, amount to the same thing.* How could this relate to what is conventionally called 'yoga' – the various techniques practised under this label?

» Īśvara is the ideal of the Right (doing, choosing). The God of the Theist, in contrast, is usually depicted as ideally Good (in character, power, and ability). Given this distinction, which we shall return to, how might devotion to Īśvara differ from devotion to the Theist's God?

» Do we gain something by thinking about Yoga or yoga as spiritual or religious? Do we lose something by denying this?

» Given that 'Yoga' is part of Hinduism because the British decided that being Indigenously Indian was a religion, how can we responsibly deal with this now? Is denying the Hindu-ness of Yoga different or the same as denying someone's racial categorization, which was also a function of external colonial decisions? Is claiming to be colour-blind (where race is concerned) wrong? If so, would being religion-blind where Yoga is concerned also be wrong?

» Given that Yoga was originally philosophy, it is a mistake to infer that we cannot practise yoga as *āsana* or some other technique. Were you concerned by the idea that Yoga is primarily philosophy? If so, or if not, why?

» What would it be like to give up on believing and instead think in terms of reasoning? How might this practice involve devotion to Īśvara?

» If you are in a YTT, are you aware of the ethics requirements for yoga teaching in your programme? What are they?

CHAPTER 2

WESTERN SAMSKĀRA-S – WESTERN COLONIALISM

saṃskāra-sākṣāt-karaṇāt pūrva-jāti-jñānam

By actively inspecting interpretive practices, past lives are revealed.

Yoga Sūtra III.18

INTRODUCTION

Expertise is an excellence in knowing: it is the ability to sort through a controversy in a specific area of inquiry. *Authority* is more ordinary: it is the power to enforce an opinion. A *saṃskāra* is an implementation of our own authority to impose an opinion on ourselves *as though* that counts as expertise.

Yoga practice has an important effect of getting us to renounce our *saṃskāra*-s. *Saṃskāra*-s don't announce themselves. They are silent mechanisms that have to be rendered explicit. A *saṃskāra* hides itself by bringing 'order' to our lives and then all we notice is the order it brings, but it is an order that undermines our autonomy and our need to be unconservative and self-governing. It is an order brought about by prejudice and habit, not responsibility.

Most people today have Western *saṃskāra*-s – especially people who descend from BIPOC areas that have been colonized by the *West* and people who inherit the *West* as their ancestral heritage. That's pretty much everyone who is human today. In popular literature, '*saṃskāra*' is a positive thing. The

Monier-Williams Sanskrit-English Dictionary[1] lists its meanings as including: putting together, forming well, making perfect, training, education; correctness; making sacred, hallowing, consecration. In Yoga, attention is brought to the ways in which a practice of 'putting together', 'forming well', 'making perfect', 'training', 'education', 'correctness', 'making sacred', 'hallowing', 'consecration' – a *saṃskāra* – institutes a repetitive practice that automates a propositional attitude, like belief, fear, or hope. This automation of a belief and other propositional attitudes as a means of informing, educating, or organizing ourselves or others is an interpretation. When we institute a *saṃskāra* we misuse our own authority over ourselves and others to impose a propositional attitude as though that imposition constitutes knowledge. As it prioritizes authority over expertise, it is a force that has no independent check. This process confuses the *precision* (the repeatability of a measure) of our beliefs with *accuracy* (the quality of being objectively true) of our outlook. *Saṃskāra*-s are precise, and not accurate. This is an ignorance, which creates a (false) sense of self (*asmitā*) that is literally dependent on one's own preferences (*sva rasa*) (YS II.6–9). In my translation of the *Yoga Sūtra*, I used the more evocative 'tendency impression' as the translation for '*saṃskāra*': interpretive practice is more explicit. This ritualization of belief explains or rather undergirds *confirmation bias*: a tendency to find what we are looking for.

For instance, if as a child, I was bitten by a dog, I can decide that either: (a) that event was an oddity and does not define me or dogs, and nothing can really be generalized about the event, or (b) dogs are scary because they bite, and I'm a person scared of dogs. The first option is what logic (Yoga) would lead us to: a sample size of one event and one perspective (mine) is too small to draw any generalizations. Logic would counsel us not to give this isolated data point much weight. The second option isn't really true: not all dogs bite, and at the time of the incident I might not have even been scared of dogs. But afterwards, I might try to assimilate and bring order to the event by creating a *saṃskāra* via the second option, and then I view every circumstance through the frame of this *saṃskāra*. If I ever happen upon a dog again, it will trigger this *saṃskāra* and deliver the judgement and visceral experience of my fear of dogs. Moreover, it creates an illusion of me being a person scared of dogs. And this visceral experience in turn seems to confirm my *saṃskāra* – if I am not critical of my role in all of this. Because of this experience, I end up reaffirming the *saṃskāra* of dog-fear – when, in reality, this experience of dog-fear is largely a creation of the *saṃskāra*. And yet, if we look at this *saṃskāra* in detail, we will learn something about the history that made it possible. If it's my *saṃskāra*, I will learn that at some point, I related to some dog(s) and decided to identify with a fear of dogs. In effect, to understand the history of this *saṃskāra* is to understand the choices involved in creating the *saṃskāra*.

Saṃskāra-s and memories are closely related (YS IV.9). A memory (*smṛti*) is an experience that we would lose if it were not for our effort to hold on to it (YS I.11). *Saṃskāra*-s (interpretations) provide the structure that allows us to hold memories as part of an effort at self-understanding. This is our baggage: this is how we are haunted by trauma. Worse, this conflation of ourselves with data of experience hides its history. We end up believing it (like my dog-fear), and then we use such beliefs to further construct a life around these beliefs. In this manner we promulgate a life that perpetuates this *kleśa* (affliction) (YS II.3). To get rid of the grip that *saṃskāra*-s have on us is to undo our own grip on ourselves, and this involves appreciating the history of a *saṃskāra* – and this is knowable by inspecting the *saṃskāra*.

In the next section, we shall review the history of the *West*, briefly. The point of this exercise is to appreciate the ways in which LAT, the most basic of the *West's saṃskāra*-s, has had a lasting influence on the course of human history. Without bringing LAT to the fore, it seems that the series of events that punctuate the *West* is a string of accidents. But this series of events involves the colonial incursion into BIPOC traditions that are then appropriated by the *West*.

In the third section, we will move on to examine how *Western saṃskāra*-s structure the contemporary discourse around yoga. One such *saṃskāra* is what is sometimes called 'modern yoga' or 'modern postural yoga'. This is a defining feature of what I shall call 'Yogaland'. With our unfolding logical skills, we see that these are severed limbs and that they are examples of *Western* Appropriated Culture (*WAC*). *WAC* is a *Western saṃskāra*. It's not Yoga, but it uses South Asian words, ideas, and cultural resources (like 'yoga') to reinstate and replicate the *Western* tradition. It is hence a deep and stealth version of colonialism. The goals, aspirations, and pedagogy of *WAC* are all *Western*. Not only are they geographically from Europe, they are also a fruition of the colonizing tradition that is the *West*. As colonialism is not good for anyone, as it involves undermining personal Sovereignty, it's bad for all concerned. *WAC* is only South Asian in so far as the appropriated cultural resources used to articulate *WAC* are South Asian. There is much to say about this topic, which we will visit throughout this book. But to begin with, we will note that there is nothing objective (reasonable, logical, rational) about *W*AC-ky severed limbs: it's interpretation all the way down.

In the fourth section, I consider some objections to the idea that the *W*AC modes of explaining yoga are foreign to the South Asian tradition.

In concluding this chapter, we will consider the ethical basis of so much of the *W*est and how the assumed ethical theory of *W*AC-ky presentations is the opposite of Yoga. This will prepare our exploration for basic ethical theory in Chapter 3, of which Yoga is an important and neglected contribution.

THE *WEST*: A BRIEF HISTORY

In this section, we will explore how LAT constitutes a *saṃskāric* backdrop to the *W*est and its colonialism. Like all *saṃskāra*-s, LAT hides itself by changing the subject. To understand how it hides itself, let us review the relationship between LAT and belief.

As what we assert in language is typically our beliefs, LAT conflates thought with belief. This converts explanations in terms of thought into explanations in terms of beliefs, which is to interpret. If I want to communicate my belief that it is raining outside, I just say, 'It is raining outside.' Speaking is largely a tool to articulate our point of view, and conflating thought with speech leads to the conflation of thought with belief: interpretation. LAT is hence a theory of thought that supports *saṃskāra*-s (instituted interpretations) as a method of explanation. As this is the basic theoretical commitment of the *W*est, the *W*est is a tradition of *saṃskāra*-s.

A *saṃskāra* is entirely circular: as it is a method of authority, it at best supports and justifies itself by enforcing itself. In the *W*estern tradition, this circularity is sometimes valorized as the *hermeneutic circle* – the inescapability of circularity in understanding. Thinkers in this tradition such as Heidegger and Gadamer acknowledge the role that language plays in mediating this circularity. In South Asia, and with traditions associated with Yoga, this circularity is called *saṃsāra* – the whirlpool – which was how ordinary, excruciating life was characterized. Yoga, which relies not on beliefs but on making options clear, shows that it is the *saṃskāra* that creates experiences that are then treated as evidence for the *saṃskāra*. Further, this shows the ways in which *saṃskāra*-s are based on irresponsible choices, which create a political reality that is our choice and for which there is no independent evidence. In short, there is no independent evidence for being scared of dogs independently of the choice to view dogs as scary. And there is no evidence for viewing dogs as scary independently of the choice to be scared of dogs. Not taking seriously our moral responsibility to choose leads us to create *saṃskāra*-s that we return to again and again (*Gītā* 9.3).

These considerations help us see that not only is interpretation the kernel of *saṃskāra*-s, in so far as interpretation arises from LAT, and languages are shared cultural resources, interpretation from LAT is a kind of groupthink and project of social conformity.

LAT is found in other traditions. While originally absent from the South Asian tradition, it is affirmed in the Chinese tradition by Confucius in the *Analects* (13.3). Many of the same political outcomes we find in the *W*est are found in the Chinese tradition too – especially authoritarianism. (China also has Taoism, which savages LAT – and so that tradition is more complex.) While LAT is *the* theme of *W*estern philosophy from its very ancient start to contemporary iterations in Analytic and Continental philosophy, LAT is a *saṃskāra* that is not simply accepted but acclaimed. It is part of the groupthink of the *W*estern tradition. I discovered this accidentally while conducting extensive PhD research on the philosophy of language. LAT is so basic, there are no alternatives in the *W*estern tradition. In addition to supporting groupthink, the emphasis on language leads to anthropocentrism, the prioritization of humans, but also the bias toward those in one's language group – one's community. But as understanding is then confused with being part of one's community, to understand others requires forcing them to be part of one's community: colonialism. As this groupthink begins in the *W*est, as it grows it treats its groupthink as though it's the universal order and everything that deviates as something to be controlled by further *saṃskāra*-s. This ugly side of LAT as a *saṃskāra* is on display when we review the murder of Socrates and the subsequent developments of the *W*est.

Ancient Greece

We know about Socrates by way of what others have said about him and the way others depicted him. Socrates was Plato's teacher, and Plato, perhaps *the most influential W*estern philosopher, never wrote anything in his own name. He ran a Philosophy school, the *Academy*, and wrote dialogues – featuring his teacher, Socrates. These dialogues split into two camps. The early dialogues depict Socrates as someone who engages, at least partly, in explication. The latter dialogues seem to articulate Plato's ideas.

The first step of explication is to derive from a perspective, via logic, a theory that entails its controversial claims. The second step is to collate those controversial claims and understand the topic in terms of what the dissenting theories disagree about. Socrates is depicted in Plato's early dialogues as attempting to implement the first step of explication with anyone he ran into: he would try to derive from what they said a theory (usually in the form of a definition) that would explain their controversial claims. Philosophy for Socrates was his way of relating to others. These early dialogues chronicle Socrates' life and his death at the hands of the Athenian Court.

Socrates' practice of Philosophy, which ended up revealing those he interacted with as shams, earned him many enemies. As reported in Plato's *Apology*, the aristocrats of Athens who felt humiliated by Socrates brought him up on the charges of: (a) promoting false gods, and (b) corrupting the youth. Just to be clear, the crime that Socrates was being charged with was, in effect, the failure to socially conform to the prevailing values of the day. This is an entailment of the *saṃskāra*, LAT. This is an important detail to keep track of when we compare the *W*est with the ancient South Asian tradition, where no one bought LAT and hence people were generally open to Philosophy as a means of inquiry. Philosophers as independent thinkers were celebrated in South Asia – philosophers such as the *Upaniṣadic* sages, the Buddha, Mahāvīra, and Kṛṣṇa (the incarnation of Viṣṇu who delivers a moral philosophy lecture on a battlefield). In South Asia, no one expected that a thinker had to answer to social expectations. In fact, as with much Philosophy, ordinary social expectations were typically scrutinized by philosophers in South Asia. Indeed, the Vedic tradition, which culminates in discussions of Yoga, is a tradition of being critical of its own social practices, moving slowly away from practices of sacrifices to the gods of nature to emphasizing the responsibility of the self. Buddhists and Jains engaged in criticizing ordinary social practices of the day, rooted in violence toward nonhuman animals. These thinkers were not brought up on charges of failing to conform to social expectations, because in the philosophical world of South Asia, the live question, in opposition to the Athenian Court, was: what gods should we worship and how should we raise the youth?

Socrates, in contrast, was made to answer for why he didn't live up to social expectations, and he did this by refuting the charges brought against him. In court, Socrates defends himself by getting an accuser to redefine (a) as the charge that he believes in no gods at all, which Socrates denies. With respect to (b), he asks his well-wishers in attendance, who he had mentored, whether he had corrupted them, and none would affirm this. Socrates might have got off, but he finishes his defence as recorded in Plato's *Apology* by claiming that if he were given the choice of exile and doing Philosophy or staying in Athens and not doing Philosophy, he would choose neither. Socrates claims that he is, in fact, doing everyone else a favour by accosting random Athenians and engaging them in philosophical conversation and should be supported by Athens. Socrates is sentenced to death. In a subsequent dialogue, the *Crito*, Socrates is given an opportunity to escape but he refuses to on the basis of three reasons: (a) the state is like his parent, (b) the state has been his benefactor, and (c) he has an agreement with the state to abide by its laws. This is worth noting. For though Socrates was a philosopher, in the end there was something oddly *W*estern about his commitment to being bound by social expectations. Also, for our purposes, it is worth noting the way in which Socrates martyrs himself for Philosophy. Martyrdom plays *no* role in Yoga or the ancient South Asian tradition.

After Socrates' death, Plato imagines an alternative universe where it is the philosopher, Socrates, who is in charge. He explores this in the *Republic*, which begins with Socrates being forced into socialization with a group of young men under threat of force. Socrates 'agrees' to join the group and then takes control by changing the topic of conversation to justice. Socrates reasons that justice in the soul and the state are the same. ('*Soul*' is a word for the mind, and since Plato, in the *W*est, you are the same as your mind. So it is often used as the translation for the Indic ideas of self – *ātmā* – but in South Asia, the mind was generally treated as something extraneous to the self.) Plato via Socrates in the *Phaedo* (81e–82e) depicts the body as a prison of the soul and states that ultimately our greatest good involves leaving and transcending the body and its sensations via Philosophy. In the *Republic*, Plato through Socrates argues that just as the soul has three parts – reason, spirit, and desire – so too must the state have three isomorphic castes. Justice in both cases occurs when reason dominates the other two components. In the state, the spirited caste are administrators of the state, and the lowest caste are the workers. The reasoning component in the state is the philosopher king who uses the light of the Good – a higher power, indeed the highest power – to appreciate abstract objects of reason. Most importantly, it is the philosopher king who sets the curriculum for the entire society. Ordinary citizens begin education at the very bottom. Those who show that they are able to master the curriculum can move up the organizational ladder of society as set up by the administrators and the philosopher king. Plato appreciates that it will be difficult to get everyone to buy into this caste system and to work to a common end. So he claims that part of the educational system, comprised of strict censorship, which even controls the kind of music people are allowed to play and listen to, will include a *Nobel Lie*: though different, we are all created by the same loving God to do our various life purposes (the *Republic* 414b–415d).

There are certain important features of Plato's vision in the *Republic*. First, radical inequality that *defines who we are* is normal. This stands in stark opposition to Yoga and related ancient South Asian philosophies that regarded individuals as radically identical and equal at some basic level that transcends sex, caste, and species (what that level is was the point of debate). On Plato's view, this kind of radical inequality constrains our potential but is an important ingredient of social cohesion. As we are defined by our mind, those of us with a troubled mind will be troubled eternally (*Phaedrus* 246a–254e). Some of us are better off following, while others are natural leaders. Second, in Plato's vision, there is no distinction or line between the *authority* to implement a curriculum and the expertise that allows us to discover what knowledge is. Socrates does claim that the guy at the top will have to be forced (the *Republic* 473d4, 500d4, 519e4, 520a8, 520e2, 521b7, 539e3, 540b5) into this position of being leader, as they will have no natural interest in power. They will have to be the victim of authority too. But it is for everyone's good, and so it should be accepted. In the end, knowledge is defined as what the guy at the top says it is as determined by the people with power to install a leader, and none of us who aren't at the top are in a position to audit or verify these claims.

In Plato's defence, he never signed anything as his position; he always put words into his teacher's mouth, and the arguments for his various claims are often so bad that it seems the dialogue's actual purpose was to stimulate philosophical discussion and not be actual doctrine. However, these ideas ended up being *extremely* influential on the course of Western history. Plato articulates the pyramid structure that conflates authority (the power to enforce an opinion) and expertise, which ends up being a mainstay of the West. Hence the West is characterized by top-down political structures where leaders are also teachers of doctrine.

Aristotle, in contrast, did leave us documents that were in his own words, but often they are not so different from Plato's. Aristotle, like Plato, claims that ethics is *political science*, or the science of getting along in one's polis (city). And like Plato, he claims that unless one has had sufficient exposure to a curriculum, one is not qualified to comment on it. And so Aristotle claims that in order for us to be able to talk about ethics, we have to have the right upbringing (*Ethics* I.3). However, like Plato, he didn't believe that most people have the capacity to engage in this reflection. Some are naturally born slaves, who would be lucky to find a master who tells them what to do (*Politics* 1.1254b).

Aristotle also departs from Plato in claiming that all of nature aims at an end (*PA* i.I.), and all pursuits aim at some good (*Ethics* I.1). In short, the way things ought to be is pretty much how they turn out naturally. This coupled with his view that moral reasoning is something we can only engage in once we have knowledge of the topic from upbringing leads him to describe the political subjection of women to men as appropriate. (Plato in the *Republic* was, in contrast, radical: he thought women and men, though generally different, should be treated and judged as individuals.) In the case of the humans that Aristotle was concerned about, the good end of life was happiness, well-being, or fulfilment (*eudaimonia*). Ethical activity then aims at these ends.

Both Plato's and Aristotle's emphasis on moral knowledge as a matter of community upbringing is an outcome of the *saṃskāra* of LAT, which leads to the conflation of thinking with the communal resource of language. Plato's and Aristotle's philosophers who are in a position to elucidate the values that structure shared culture prop up the idea that communal upbringing is the foundational source of knowledge. Here, the 'logic' of the philosopher is the *logos* (language) of the community. In effect, Plato and Aristotle, both philosophers, because they took some interest in explicating a diversity of philosophical theories, articulate a view of social organization and pedagogy where Philosophy plays no role in basic learning. Rather, conformity to authority is basic – the authority of a shared cultural upbringing. These are *saṃskāra* theories of learning and are quire foreign to the Yoga tradition and the South Asian tradition. In effect, Plato and Aristotle think we need to have the right *saṃskāra*-s before we are in a position to engage in enlightened discussion. This is because we need to have the right beliefs before we are in a position to engage in enlightened conversation, and the idea that our beliefs do the explanation is a *saṃskāra* theory of knowledge.

Romans and Religion

The successors to ancient Greece were the Romans, who inherited the philosophies of Plato and Aristotle, not to mention the *West*'s LAT. With the Romans we find the authoritarianism of these earlier Platonic and Aristotelian visions taken to a globalizing political structure. Whereas Plato in Book X of the *Republic* argues that outsiders have to be kept away from the ideal city, the authoritarian solution is colonialism: forcing outsider communities to be part of one's empire. The Romans invented a term to talk about colonized, BIPOC, traditions that were tolerated within colonialism: *religio* (tradition) – religion.

Originally, the followers of Jesus were not regarded as having *religio*. On the one hand, labelling a tradition as having *religio* was a way to insulate the Roman Empire from criticism, as the position was cast as a matter of tradition, not moral and political philosophy. Yet deciding that a tradition had *religio* (as opposed to *superstitione*) was a political prize within the colonial context. Jews were apparently recognized as having *religio*, but ancient Christians were not and were instead persecuted; in time, that flipped. The Roman Emperor Constantine's conversion to Christianity and its institution as the official religion managed to further appropriate an alien tradition by making it the official position of *Western* power. Those interested in decolonization would do well to appreciate how Jesus was himself originally a victim of *Western* colonialism: it was the Romans who crucified him, as a non-Roman, BIPOC thinker and leader. Christianity, a religion that ends up blending many doctrines from Plato and Aristotle with the Gospels, is a later colonial development. But all religion is in an important sense a colonial development given that religion is just a way to classify BIPOC traditions that are tolerated by *Western* colonialism. With this, various other non-*Western*, Indigenous-but-nevertheless-European traditions were stamped out and marginalized. Europe as a largely *Western* place is a result of the colonization of Europe by the *West*. The creation of religion is the creation of *saṃskāra*-s, which are then treated as facts of who we are, and not the result of the history of oppression.

By the time Islam came about many centuries later, it inherited many of these features of the *West*, including the distinction between Philosophy (*Western* intellectual tradition) and religion. Islamic thinkers continued the conversation with *Western* philosophy and seemed to also adopt the *Western* idea of thought as speech.[2] Importantly, the idea of there being an 'official religion' had become commonplace in the *Western* tradition by this time. And hence when the British showed up in South Asia, and coined the idea of

Hinduism, it was not a stretch to reach back to the Roman idea of religion to classify South Asians as a way to normalize the subservience of the *religified* other, while also nodding to the *W*estern expectation that communities have official religions. 'Spirituality' has a history within Christian thought. Now it is increasingly used to label the same topic as religion – in English – from the twentieth century on. 'Religion' is usually reserved for the organized variety of this topic, while 'spirituality' is reserved for the non-organized, individual, variety.

British Colonization and the *W*esternization of South Asia

The way the British continued this ancient Roman project was to decide that South Asians would be tolerated as colonial subservients with their own religious identity. 'Hindu' was born of this political project to normalize the subservience of Indigenous South Asian tradition to British rule. 'Hindu' was the British way to identify the Indigenous South Asian religion that was not Islam.

South Asians as people on the receiving end of this colonial aggression reacted in various ways. Those with ancient, precolonial traditions continued to practise those. These traditions go back to a time when South Asians didn't have religious identities. They took up and defended various positions in moral philosophy with the word 'Dharma', which was their way to explore the concept of *THE RIGHT OR THE GOOD*. In Chapter 3, we will review *THE RIGHT OR THE GOOD*, which South Asians debated. One of these positions is Yoga/ Bhakti. However, as a matter of colonization, many South Asians bought the *W*estern notion of religion and then repurposed the Indigenous term 'dharma', which was used to talk about religion. Here the idea of Hinduism as *Sanātana Dharma* (the ancient or timeless Dharma) is born as a means to conceptualize Indigenous, inclusive, South Asian religion. With LAT in the background, there was a movement to distinguish between a Hindu language, written with Devanagari (what Sanskrit is often written in) – Hindi – and a Muslim language written in Arabic script – Urdu. However, it's the same language, Hindustani, and the only differences are the script it's written in and the politics of the people who speak it. Nationalism is a historically *W*estern mode of political organization usually arranged around linguistic identity. The move to create a 'Hindu' language served as the condition for the birth of Hindu Nationalism, known for Far-Right, xenophobic, and Islamophobic politics. All of these developments would be impossible without the *W*estern *saṃskāra*, LAT. And religion in particular is a most *W*estern *saṃskāra*, as it provides a way to treat the *W*est as the universal standard of humanity and then assess all other traditions in terms of their conformity to or deviation from this tradition. Spirituality is derivatively also a *W*estern *saṃskāra* that serves to prop up the centrality of the *W*est as the default, secular standard of humanity.

While this brief history starts in ancient Greece and ends in South Asia, this project of *W*estern colonialism was an expansion in all directions: hence, BIPOC traditions are rebranded as spiritual or religious, and the *W*estern tradition as secular. One reason it was so successful is that it traded on *saṃskāra*-s that hide their origins. They hide their origins for they appropriate resources of alien traditions as they spread, and if you are only looking out for cultural resources, they seem local. Without appreciating how this *saṃskāra* works to continue basic assumptions from the *W*estern tradition, it is very easy to treat these appropriative movements as mere local innovations. When, for instance, Hindus decide they need a Hindu language, it seems like a local South Asian matter as 'Hindu' just means India. When Hindus decide they have a religion, Hinduism, it seems local. When it looks like they have this practice that focuses on posture or breathing, that seems local. When we track the spread of the *W*est via the transmission and implementation of its *saṃskāra*-s, its history is revealed as a rupture. Modern yoga, for instance, is not simply South Asian, and not simply *W*estern: it is the appropriative continuation of *W*estern colonization.

LEGITIMIZING *W*ESTERN APPROPRIATED CULTURE (*W*AC)

*W*AC is a *saṃskāra* of colonialism: it takes ideas, resources, and activities from BIPOC traditions and then employs them in service of *saṃskāra*-s from the *W*est. The very idea that *culture* is a sign of a tradition is entirely *W*estern, and Aristotelian. It arises from the *saṃskāra* of LAT. If Philosophy is the basis of the South Asian and Yoga traditions, then culture becomes an object of criticism, not the foundation of knowledge. Then, learning about the Yoga tradition is learning Philosophy. In the *W*est, tradition is identified primarily with cultural expectations, as Socrates found out the hard way. *W*estern philosophers, such as Plato and Aristotle, built on this afterwards. *W*AC continues this very *W*estern way of thinking about tradition, but by appropriating alien cultural resources as the social expectations that we are supposed to conform to. But in the process, it destroys BIPOC traditions that are built on Philosophy, not culture.

Religion

Religion is a primordial example of *W*AC. When a tradition is given a religious identity, it is no longer understood in terms of what it has to contribute to our understanding of the philosophical options. It is rather treated as something that is religious by virtue of being extraneous to the *W*estern tradition. It is hence interpreted, and this depicts the matter as one of faith and mysticism as it deviates from the beliefs of the *W*est.

However, to normalize this subservience, it is often propped up with *W*estern ideas from Plato (of the importance of top-down, doctrinal organization) and Aristotle (of the importance of cultural participation as the means to knowledge of the tradition). This leads us to interpret BIPOC traditions as though they must have some type of Platoesque-top-down, pyramid structure with a guru or central book at the top specifying a community's curriculum, or an Aristotelian-cultural-immersion in shared values requirement. This hence makes Religious Studies possible. Religious Studies employs the social sciences, such as Anthropology and Linguistics, to study the social practices of various religions and their doctrinal texts, *as though that's what is required to understand them.* As I point out, this approach to studying BIPOC traditions, and the Indian tradition especially, will provide an accurate picture of these traditions after they have been colonized by the *W*est. It will not help us understand what happened before. It is, in effect, *a*historical.

The reason religion will not help us understand what happened prior to colonization is that the very personal ideals that *W*AC ends up redeploying as religious were simply the philosophical values of contrasting ethical theories. But once we interpret these entities with our beliefs, they become mysterious, as belief is nonrational. Prior to *W*esternization, South Asians did not endorse the LAT. Hence, they were free to celebrate their philosophical values in art and not simply with words. For instance, the three action ideals of Yoga – *Īśvara praṇidhāna*, or Devotion to Sovereignty; *tapas*, or unconservatism; and *svādhyāya*, self-determination – were graphically depicted (respectively) as the Cosmic Serpent, Ādi Śeṣa, devoted to Viṣṇu (a deity depicted as distinct from his various activities, such as the disk), and Lakṣmī (depicted as a lotus who sits on herself and governs herself), floating over an ocean of external influence (the mental influences we still by our practice). When South Asians depicted these ideals, they were depicting the ideas of Yoga. Hence, the very earliest philosophical reflection on Yoga, the philosophy, mentions Viṣṇu governing the realm we enter when we practise yoga (this is a dialogue in the *Kaṭha Upaniṣad*, which we shall cover later). Viṣṇu delivers a lecture on Yoga, the moral theory, on the famous battlefield (in the *Bhagavad Gītā*) and the various stories of these three ideals are moral philosophical thought experiments about these practical values. Philosophically in the tradition, Viṣṇu is associated with Yoga/Bhakti. In contrast, Śiva is depicted as the ideal observer, and his partner Śakti (depicted in various moods) is the full content of his experiences. Śiva, in contrast, is associated with the diametrically opposed *teleological* philosophies such as Consequentialism and Virtue Ethics (we will review these theories in detail in Chapter 3). But once all of this is rendered *W*AC-ky, we do not understand these values as part of philosophical theories that entail practical conclusions. We see them as the subject of beliefs – attitudes that thoughts are true – rendering them nonrational and mysterious because belief is nonrational. It is an important part of *W*estern colonialism to hide Indigenous moral theorizing, and to depict Indigenous people as practically irrational and in need of the *W*est, which supplies moral and political wisdom. And this move to view BIPOC traditions as religious or spiritual, which is crucial to their subjugation within *W*estern colonialism, consists in projecting backwards, anachronistically, ideas and distinctions that are not Indigenous but a product of colonialism, on to the tradition.

Yogaland

In a *W*esternized world, we learn not about Yoga but about a *W*AC presentation of 'yoga'. This is called 'modern yoga' or 'modern postural yoga'. We will explore this topic in Chapter 7. But for now we can note that *W*AC yoga is a *severed limb*. *Āsana*, postural exercises, and *Prāṇāyāma*, breath work, are *ways of implementing* the philosophy of Yoga – hence they are *limbs* of Yoga. But *W*AC severs their connection to Yoga the philosophy and presents these limbs as ways to promulgate the *W*estern tradition. It is *as though W*esterners cannot help themselves. Driven by *W*estern *saṃskāra*-s they approach BIPOC traditions as raw resources to recreate *W*estern moral and political organizations.

So instead of beginning with Yoga, the philosophy, as a frame to engage in various limbs (as suggested at the very start of this book), in *W*AC-ky presentations, severed limbs are taught as the basic topic of yoga, and Philosophy is a distant concern. Here, students are introduced to Platoesque, pyramid-like yoga schools with some guru at the top who has no expertise save their authority to control the pyramid. What is typically learned is some severed limb of yoga, whether *āsana* or *prāṇāyāma*. Students see it as their job to fit into the pyramid by mastering skills, which will allow them to climb its organizational rungs. This is the Plato *saṃskāra* in Yogaland.

Or *W*AC takes an Aristotelian approach. Education of yoga is about cultural immersion in some yoga cultural values and norms, where people say 'namaste' and trot out South Asian deities as props and decorations (not as objects of devotional practice), take retreats to idyllic yoga communities as the foundation of their yoga education, or even go on trips to India to learn yoga. In this case, the yoga student tries to *go native*. The Aristotelian is motivated to change their name to something in Sanskrit or an Indic language and start wearing turbans or sarees because, on their view, it's cultural performance that is knowledge. This Aristotelianism also motivates advanced learning and training in Sanskrit and other Indic cultural practices as though that were sufficient for knowledge of yoga. (Yes, you need to learn about South Asia, including its languages, to be a researcher of Yoga, but that is not sufficient to understand Yoga on a Yoga account. You need to be a philosopher.) The goal of all of this is the practitioner's well-being and happiness. (Yoga brings about our happiness and well-being. Yoga, however, criticizes doing anything for goals as irrational. We shall explore this more in Chapter 3.) In contrast to Yoga's criticism of *prakṛti* (nature, external influence) as relevant to personal decisions, the natural is prized by the Aristotelian, and yoga is thought to be a way to celebrate the natural.

A topic of recent investigation is the space for the overlap between natural cures, such as juices, crystals, herd immunity, and a demonization of what is perceived to be unnatural, such as vaccines, even lifestyle choices, and gender and sex identities that are not interpreted as natural. Some have identified this as 'conspirituality', which combines spirituality and conspiracy theorizing. According to the original definition, this consists of two commitments: '1) a secret group covertly controls, or is trying to control, the political and social order, and 2) humanity is undergoing a "paradigm shift" in consciousness.'[3] What students of the history of Philosophy will note is that what makes conspirituality possible is an Aristotelian *saṃskāra*, which assumes that things are defined by some natural end, which is good, and what departs from this supposed natural end is bad. In conspirituality, the good end, where things are going, is what requires this shift in consciousness, and the bad, the diversion from this good end, is the conspiracy. As it relies on an Aristotelian *saṃskāra*, conspirituality is a wholly *W*estern phenomenon. It also relies, fundamentally, on interpretation (also *W*estern): explanation in terms of beliefs about the requirements of spirituality and the aims of the conspiracy. And as a sign of *W*AC-kyness, conspiritualists can sometimes make use of ideas we might associate with Yoga, such as the idea that we must engage in personal transformation to be in tune with the requirements of spirituality. Often, a quote attributed to M. K. Gandhi (that we must *be the change* we want to see) is thrown into the mix. But this is *W*AC-ky. In Yoga, conspiracy theorizing is absent. In Yoga, systemic harm occurs because we internalize the external politics we perceive as our egotism (*asmitā*). So the source of evil is not some secret group influencing us. It is our own failure to be devoted to Sovereignty, which results in our participation in systemic harm. The personal transformation Yoga requires is not private: it is public and political. We see this in Silva's example we noted in Chapter 1 of 'Racism as Self-Love'. There is no secret conspiracy that makes someone racist. It is by virtue of their internalization of the politics of White Supremacy that they become racist: that's their choice. According to Yoga, we solve problems by being responsible.

Moreover, according to Yoga, the construction of an ego (*asmitā*) by interpretation creates paranoia as an affliction: for then the egotist views whatever is not in conformity with the beliefs they have identified with as a personal threat. Conspiracy theorizing hence originates here, via a failure to view personal responsibility as the foundation of problem solving. And this originates via an identification with an outlook, as opposed to one's requirements to be unconservative and self-governing. So, contrary to misinformation, Yoga, the philosophy, and conspirituality have nothing in common. Yoga, the philosophy, rather explains how the paranoia of conspiracy theorizing arises out of a failure to be autonomous.

Yet, given that there are these two approaches to explanation, Yoga practitioners have an explanation for actual conspiracies: people who believe in conspiracies. We can see all of this coming to a head with the anti-science position that conspiritualists take on Covid-19. Yoga, explication, which as we shall see in Chapter 3 is about the logic-based processing of data, leads us to prefer evidence (research)-based answers to the question of what Covid-19 is and how we could be protected from the disease it causes. Social distancing, masking, and vaccines are important prophylactics as the research has shown. Conspiritualists viewed public health experts who were interested in protecting people's autonomy from illness as agents of a conspiracy. Here, the Aristotelian *saṃskāra* shines through as a preference for what is perceived to be natural (like the Covid-19 virus itself) over artificial and deliberate interventions (such as vaccines). Failure to take Covid-19 seriously has real-world consequences, like death. For Yoga, that is something to be avoided as it undermines autonomy. Conspiritualists, in contrast, treat that as preferable to artificial intervention. And their decision to undermine public health by not following evidenced-based prophylaxis against Covid-19 is conspiratorial. This highlights a general point in Yoga. A failure to be in charge of an external influence (a *vṛtti*) leads us to exemplify it. The conspiritualist, and conspirators, conspire because they are not in charge of conspiracy theorizing as an explanation. It hence influences their behaviour.

South Asians can also acquire and participate in these Platoesque or Aristotelian *saṃskāra*-s. It is, however, a sign of *WAC*-ky colonization. In both the Platonic and Aristotelian cases, learning does not begin with Philosophy, and it may never involve it at all. No one motivated by these *saṃskāra*-s regards *explicating* the options (the basic task of Philosophy) as the proper starting point.

One of the depraved outcomes of *WAC* is the plethora of teacher–student abuse scandals, where the yoga guru, at the top of a vast organization of yoga pedagogy, turns out to be a sexual predator. This has led some to observe the phenomenon of *post-lineage yoga*, where the practice of *WAC* yoga, and its severed limbs, comes apart from gurus presiding over yoga organizations. In a world of *WAC*, it seems like these problems are problems of yoga, yoga schools, and yoga teachers. But since this is *WAC*, these problems are not problems of Yoga at all. These abuses of authority are pure *WAC*.

'Academic' Legitimation of *WAC*

The 'academic' legitimation of *WAC* is systemic and a deep problem. It shows up, for instance, in the applications of colonial categories of religion and spirituality to the study of South Asian philosophy, including Yoga. It correlatively shows up in the idea that Philosophy is not the main means of studying Yoga. Rather, the main means of studying Yoga is everything aside from Philosophy, especially Ethnography and Linguistics. And this has everything to do with LAT. LAT leads *W*esterners to assume that studying 'Yoga' is about interpreting linguistic uses of 'yoga'.

If we were to explicate, we would discover that there was only one basic theory called Yoga, which concerned devotion to Īśvara and the practice of the essential traits of Sovereignty: unconservatism (*tapas*) and self-governance (*svādhyāya*). We would also render explicit that there were many implementations of this practice, also called yoga, such as the limbs, and that these limbs were appropriated by other philosophical theories. What changes, if anything, are the flavours and the contours of the limbs, but the basic philosophical theory – Yoga – that motivates these various limbs is abstract and unchanging. But if we were to adopt LAT, which motivates *W*AC, we would treat each reference to a limb of yoga as a unique definition of yoga. And hence, over time, the number of different flavours of various limbs of yoga would multiply, and we might even end up concluding, absurdly, that yoga has changed and evolved into 'modern yoga'. One could not draw the conclusion that yoga has changed and evolved except by confusing linguistic behaviour around what people use 'yoga' for, with Yoga. The conclusion that yoga has changed because what people use 'yoga' for has changed is like concluding that mice have changed, for now the word 'mouse' is used not only for a kind of mammal but also for input devices for personal computers.

In the case of Yoga, the various uses of 'yoga' can easily be explained as an entailment of the basic philosophy of Yoga. But if we ignore logic and explication and instead interpret 'yoga' on the basis of what people call yoga via LAT, then we can create a field called 'Yoga Studies' – dominated by philologists and ethnographers, who study the linguistic behaviour of people's use of the word 'yoga'. Imagine if we did the same for vaccines. We could create 'Vaccine Studies', which would be a field devoted to people's opinions about vaccines and their use of the word 'vaccine'. We could also take a philological approach: study all the things historically people have written about vaccines. While certainly there is value in studying things like vaccine hesitancy, or popular and historical opinions about vaccines, that's quite different from studying vaccines. If there were no difference, then people's opinions about vaccines would be the same as vaccines. But they aren't. Similarly, while we can study people's beliefs about yoga and their use of the word 'yoga', that is quite different from studying Yoga. The discipline we would need to engage in for the study of Yoga is Philosophy. Philosophy, recall, is not compatible with colonialism, and hence it is displaced in colonial discussions of Yoga by *W*AC and the study of Platoesque and Aristotelian *saṃskāra*-s as though that is studying Yoga.

OBJECTION: SOUTH ASIANS ARE LIKE THIS TOO!

*W*AC normalizes *W*estern colonialism. One startling outcome of this normalization is that when we learn about South Asia, say about religion, or yoga, we're really learning *W*AC, which is an active colonialism. Especially in Yogaland, the obsession with lineages or communities for the practice of yoga as though that were a requirement for learning about yoga is entirely *W*estern. One might object to this by claiming that *South Asians have their own Indigenous lineages and communities. Lineages and communities were not invented by the West but are part of human social interaction. So what we find in modern yoga is in fact a simple continuity of Indigenous lineages and yoga-centred cultural experiences.*

Answering this objection requires care to pay attention to history. It also involves being careful to stick to the Yogic values of *ahiṃsā*, which disrupts systemic harm, like Islamophobia. On a Yoga account, ethical practice is a matter of solidarity with people. Religious identity doesn't define who we are: it is a creation of *W*estern colonization. Yogic practice involves appreciating all of our common interest in our own unconservatism and self-governance, which means creating spaces for diverse peoples with diverse backgrounds to participate in their own independence. Hence, Yoga entails a sharp rebuke of bigotry. A person's religious identity tells us nothing about who they are, on a Yogic account, and so we should give everyone an opportunity to figure that out for themselves. Moreover, as we shall see, Yoga entails that each one of us as devotees of Īśvara is responsible for the values that we adopt. Yoga the philosophy allows people to choose those values, which may be of, say, Muslim or Christian origin. We shall look at this in Chapter 3 (and explain how, for instance, there is a way that one could be a Christian Yogi and a way one could not).

However, *W*estern colonization in South Asia begins when the rulers themselves understand the possibilities in terms of the *W*est and its colonial notions, such as religion, and the earliest example of this *W*estern colonialism is the Delhi Sultanate. This is a Muslim empire (1206–1526), with origins outside of South Asia. This begins centuries of colonial rule in South Asia, which is then taken over by the British. Traditions that *predate* the origins of

*W*estern colonization in South Asia are our link to what South Asia was like *prior* to being overrun by *W*AC.

If we look at precolonial, Indigenous, South Asian Yoga, it is an activity that happens *within Philosophy* which involves abandoning the circularity of *saṃskāra*-s. This means that in the Indigenous case of Yoga, the primary topic to be taught is Philosophy, and the limbs of Yoga are presented as supports for the philosophical practice of Yoga/Bhakti as a basic ethical theory. Moreover, an important part of the Yoga tradition is a rejection of the LAT-informed expectation that knowledge begins with groupthink and the sharing of community-wide values. In traditions associated with Yoga, such as Buddhism and Jainism, we see the founders leaving ordinary society to pursue philosophical experimentation and ultimately to settle on their chosen philosophical practice. The counterculture nature of Yoga/Bhakti is celebrated in stories of exemplary Yogis who are children or young teens, who in various ways break with ordinary culture. This list includes Nāciketa (about whom we will learn in Chapter 6), Namāḻvār, Prahlāda, Dhruva, and Āṇḍāḷ.

Namāḻvār (perhaps 700 CE) is especially illustrative of this trend. He is the child Yogi who is the first human in the lineage of Śrī Vaiṣṇava teachers. Krishnamacharya, often regarded by *W*AC as the father of modern yoga (who taught many influential yoga teachers), was a Śrī Vaiṣṇava.

According to legend, Namāḻvār was serene to the point of being unresponsive from birth. His parents didn't know what to do with him so they left him at the foot of a tamarind tree at a Viṣṇu (*tapas*) temple, where he meditated. In time, the brightness of this practice attracted an elderly Yogi, Madhurakavi, who became the child's first devotee. And so began the lineage of human Śrī Vaiṣṇava teachers: the first being a child Yogi from birth, whose first student is a full-grown man. Moreover, Namāḻvār was reportedly a member of the *Vellalar*, agricultural caste (which according to prescriptive views on caste from Brahmanical literature would make him a *Śūdra*, which is regarded as the lowest of four castes), while Madhurakavi was a Brahmin, which is often regarded as the highest of castes. The next teacher in this lineage is not Madhurakavi, but Nāthamuni, who tradition records as an accomplished Yogi himself. He learned from Namāḻvār not by direct contact or receiving teaching but by meditating on Namāḻvār. Āṇḍāḷ, a female teenager, is also venerated in this tradition as the goddess Lakṣmī (self-determination) herself. In her explicit poetry (the *Nāciyār Tirumoḻi*) she relates sexually and romantically to Viṣṇu, against social norms and expectations of men (including her father).

She comes to be known as 'Āṇḍāḷ', which means *the one who rules* (she gets her way).

What is important about these stories is that they are a celebration of yogic practice as something that we *choose* to do and which is not in any way a function of upbringing, authority, special education, access to something uncommon, or caste status. Contrary to Plato, Aristotle, and Western *saṃskāra*-s based on LAT, which value and promote groupthink and enculturation, according to Yoga, age and experience is not a condition of Yoga, for it is simply our choice to be devoted to Īśvara, which breaks down into *tapas* (unconservatism) and *svādhyāya* (self-governance). It is this choice to be devoted to Īśvara that is the initiation and the fruition of our practice of Yoga. Such stories encode how Yoga is not about patriarchy (which involves the prioritization of the older over the younger or men over women). Namāḻvār, the unenculturated, low-caste child, becomes the teacher of all subsequent Śrī Vaiṣṇava, and Āṇḍāḷ, an exemplar of self-determination choosing unconservatism (*tapas*) as her value and determining her own sexuality against conventional expectations.

The example of Nāthamuni learning from a teacher he has no direct contact with is much like what we are doing. We are working on our yogic skill of explication to learn from Patañjali and other philosophers from the past. And this is made possible by putting Philosophy first. This also contrasts with the Platoesque and Aristotelian *saṃskāra*-s of Yogaland, where knowledge is passed down by contact with teachers *as though students can't do their own learning themselves.* In the West, via LAT, 'learning' is retooled into the social transmission of interpretations.

As South Asia becomes colonized by Western rulers, things change and, in time, all of the *saṃskāra*-s of the West, including the Plato and Aristotle *saṃskāra*-s, as well as LAT, religion, and nationalism, become the norm. But if we inspect the history of these *saṃskāra*-s, we can choose not to participate in Western colonization.

YOGA IS ABOUT YOU, NOT WHO YOU KNOW

I have chosen the acronym *WAC* on purpose. It highlights the way in which so much of what people with Western *saṃskāra*-s take to be Indigenous and BIPOC is itself an absurd continuation of the West. All of this is hence WAC-ky. I've also chosen to deliberately call what is taught within contexts of *WAC* in 'yoga' spaces *severed limbs*. They are literally the limbs of Yoga severed from the original moral philosophical practice. Calling the appropriated practice from Yoga severed limbs brings attention to the ways in which it is violent, and it is hence part of the violence of colonialism. It is violent as it destroys knowledge and understanding of Yoga. It encourages and supports the *saṃskāra* of LAT, which permits each severed limb to be its own yoga. It replicates colonial expectations while hiding its politics.

An important commonality of Plato and Aristotle as theorists of LAT is their commitment to Virtue Ethics. Virtue Ethics claims that the right thing to do is what the virtuous agent would want, and if you yourself are not virtuous, you ought to find someone who is to tell you what to do. This version of Virtue Ethics cements the authoritarian structure of *WAC* severed limbs, whether in its Platoesque or Aristotelian versions. Yoga, the basic moral and political theory, takes the opposite view. Figuring out what to do is the job of each one of us and cannot be foisted on someone else. By being devoted to Sovereignty, Īśvara, we are doing the right thing. And as we perfect this practice of right choosing and doing independently, our behaviour becomes good and beneficial to ourselves and others. The key to this is taking on the practice of being devoted to Īśvara, which consists in being devoted to unconservatism and self-governance. Other people can be a support to us: they can even be our teachers, facilitating a space and access to information for us to do our own work. But our work, like eating or resting, is ours to do ourselves. So whereas *saṃskāra*-s keep us conservatively stuck in some perspective, and prevent us from revisiting choices and decisions, the practice of Yoga is the opposite. To understand this we have to explicate the options.

CHAPTER 2 REFLECTIONS

» Now that you have been introduced to the idea of a *saṃskāra*, can you identify *saṃskāra*-s that have defined your life?

» Can you observe the history of your own *saṃskāra*-s?

» Are you *WAC*-ky?

» If you were 'introduced' to yoga as a practice of *WAC*-ky severed limbs, how could you correct your practice?

- What does starting with Philosophy, before a severed limb, look like? Can you put into effect the framing exercise introduced in Chapter 1 to contextualize your practice of yoga?
- What would it take for you to engage in a practice of Yoga as opposed to severed limbs?
- Is your introduction to yoga Aristotelian or Platonistic in any way?
- How does Yoga help us fight Islamophobia and other forms of bigotry while also appreciating history and the actions of agents with various identity markers?
- When you think of a Yoga guru, do you think of someone like Namāḻvār or Āṇḍāḷ – people who did their own thing? Or do you think of someone who tells you what to do?
- As we explore the precolonial basis of Yoga, and the colonial, what *saṃskāra*-s come to the surface?

CHAPTER 3

YOGA AS A BASIC ETHICAL (DHARMA) THEORY

Over the last 2500 years, Western philosophers have formed three main theories on how to live an ethical life. First of all there is Virtue Ethics... Aristotle believed that there were certain virtues of mind and character like courage or generosity and you should try to develop yourself in accordance with those virtues. Next there is Consequentialism. The basis for judgment of whether something is right or wrong stems from the consequences of that action... And finally there is Deontology... being ethical is about identifying...duties and following those rules... But here's the thing my chili babies: all three of those theories are hot stinking cat dookie. The true meaning of life is – the actual system that you should all follow is – Nihilism. The world is empty, there is no point to anything, and you're just going to die. So do whatever!! And now I am going to eat my marshmallow, candy chili in silence and you can jump up your own butts.

Prof. Chidi Anagonye, 'Jeremy Bearimy', 3.4 *The Good Place*

INTRODUCTION

Being a philologist, linguist, ethnographer, or historian *does not disqualify you* from talking about Yoga. Also, these skills *do not qualify* one to speak with any authority or expertise on Philosophy in general and Yoga, the philosophy, in particular. Really, this should go without saying. Being a dentist does not, by virtue of being a dentist, provide any knowledge of what an Indian philosopher has to say, even though an Indian philosopher uses their mouth and teeth to articulate their views. Similarly, being a Sanskritist does not provide any knowledge, by virtue of being a Sanskritist, about Indian philosophy, even though Indian philosophers such as Patañjali used Sanskrit to articulate their views. And yet, in a world dominated by the *W*est, where interpretation reigns, it's not disciplinary knowledge that counts but relatable opinions. And given LAT at the start of this tradition (in its idea of *logos*) the linguist is the dilettante that gets top billing. And let's face it: in this climate of *W*AC-kyism, *W*AC-ky people do not want to learn about Philosophy. They want to feel unthreatened in the idea that their opinions are perfect and wonderful. Prioritizing Linguistics and not Philosophy allows a whole swathe of dilettante academics and dilettante 'students' of Yoga to avoid the hard work of learning Philosophy, which is at the heart of the South Asian tradition. Ironically, the more 'teaching' and 'research' on Yoga is focused on South Asian culture and language, the less anyone is actually engaging with this tradition.

But more importantly, even merely being a philosopher is required to understand what South Asian thinkers had to say about philosophical matters – but it's not enough. A philosopher is someone who explicates the options on topics that are defined by their controversy and then provides reasons for their choices. This is a big requirement, and some *W*estern academics, especially those hired to teach South Asian philosophy, fail to meet it given the privilege they derive and rely on from the *W*estern tradition – a privilege that in many cases got them the job. University Philosophy departments are often staffed with people who participate in *W*estern interpretation and they would sooner hire someone who does the same. But assuming that one is a philosopher who can and does explicate, explicating the philosophical options of BIPOC traditions requires more learning than most philosophers do. It requires being a philosopher but also gaining linguistic, cultural, and historical knowledge of a BIPOC tradition. I suppose this is the confusing part to the uncritical: they observe the need to be familiar with the language of South Asian philosophy to read its texts and confuse that with the expertise necessary to understand the text. That's like observing that philosophers need to eat breakfast to have energy to read a text in the morning, and then confusing the eating of breakfast with the expertise required to understand a text. If you are starving, you will not be able to understand Philosophy. But it doesn't follow that being well fed is what constitutes understanding Philosophy. One can be hungry and understand Philosophy.

Most philosophers are simply trained in the *W*estern tradition and hence lack knowledge of what lies beyond. And as this tradition generates and supports interpretation as part of its ancient model of thought, it takes a fair bit of philosophical discipline to rise above these cultural predilections to appreciate what philosophical questions boil down to. One can easily float in a *W*esternized world by way of *W*estern *saṃskāra*-s. Most philosophers do not engage in the deeper work and mistake the views that they are familiar with for the extent of a topic. So instead of explicating what basic ethical theories entail, philosophers in the *W*estern tradition conflate a theory, like say Virtue Ethics, with what a famous *W*estern Virtue Ethicist (like Aristotle) says. And the result is an experience of despair because the options are so restrictive. The epigraph above is a great example of how restricting one's study of the options to the *W*estern tradition leads to both the conflation of understanding theories with famous *W*estern versions and despair. Why? According to the Yoga tradition, focusing on these three ethical theories will lead to despair because they have one problem in common: they define the right thing to do in terms of the good. That means that when things are bad – exactly when we need help – these theories have nothing to offer.

Yoga is a fourth basic ethical theory in addition to the familiar three: Virtue Ethics, Consequentialism, and Deontology. Yoga, in contrast to these three, defines the right thing to do in terms of the ideal of the Right (Īśvara). So even when things are bad, we can work on doing right, and devotion to that, in time and with practice, turns our activity into success. With Yoga, we can always be optimistic.

In this chapter, we shall do some preparatory work to understand how Yoga, among the basic ethical theories, is unique in its capacity to save us from despair. But more importantly, we shall explore *how* Yoga is a basic ethical theory.

Understanding the importance of Yoga involves understanding the importance of the rich history of South Asian moral philosophy, which is exactly what *W*AC-ky discourse and 'scholarship' wants to avoid. It needs to avoid this topic because explicating the South Asian options requires that we put aside our *saṃskāra*-s and *W*AC-ky prejudices to learn from the South Asian tradition. This upsets *W*estern colonialism and the assumed privilege the *W*est has in explaining everything. When we study South Asian moral (dharma) philosophy, it's the *West* that is revealed for its historical peculiarities.

In the next section, we will begin by reviewing some of the basics of logic, which we need to explicate, but which are important aspects of Yoga, the basic philosophical practice. Logic is Yoga. In the third section, we will then apply these logical skills to rendering explicit four basic ethical theories, of which Yoga is one. Yoga is unique among options in that understanding Yoga allows you to understand *all* the options. In the fourth section we will consider the history of the development of Yoga and review many South Asian positions that are related to Yoga and confused with Yoga. Finally, we will conclude with some reflections on how Yoga is the ethics that we require for practising and teaching Yoga.

LOGIC AND YOGA

The *Yoga Sūtra* (YS I.2) begins with the definition of Yoga as *citta-vṛt-ti-nirodhaḥ*. In the next chapter, we will explore in depth the many important meanings in this definition of Yoga. But one important meaning is the idea of yoga as an activity of checking and influencing, what follows from what we can contemplate. This is an important aspect of Yoga, as this is essentially logic.

Logic has to do with the support that data, including thoughts, can supply to other thoughts. The support that data and thoughts can supply to other thoughts is independent of whether the data or thoughts are true or reliable. Importantly, putting together arguments that exemplify the virtues of reason (inferential support) is work and involves checking and influencing the data and thoughts so that they take on a reasonable form. And this reasonable form protects and respects our own individuality as knowers: nothing in this organization requires that we believe or buy what we are organizing. But the output of this organizational work is knowledge of what is organized. Hence, the result is, as the *Yoga Sūtra* (YS I.2) describes: *tadā draṣṭuḥ svarūpe'vasthānam* – then the seer (knower) can abide in its essence.

There are three basic forms of logic. We have familiarized ourselves with one of them: deduction. Deduction is a kind of argument that is comprised of some thoughts that are reasons (premises) and another thought that is the conclusion. Ideally, the reasons should support the conclusion. This occurs when the argument is logically *valid*. A valid deductive argument is an argument where if the premises are true, the conclusion has to be true. To keep things simple, let us return to our examples from Chapter 1:

Premise 1: The Moon is a squash.
Premise 2: Squashes grow on trees.
Conclusion: The Moon grows on a tree.

Everything said here is false. However, if the two premises are true, the conclusion has to be true. Valid arguments can be comprised of entirely false propositions, like this one. And then there was the other example of an invalid argument with true propositions:

Premise 1: Biden was POTUS in 2021.
Premise 2: Modi was PM of India in 2021.
Conclusion: Shyam Ranganathan is the author of this book.

These examples serve to distinguish truth from logic. Some people brainwashed by the *W*estern tradition hold that understanding is always an explanation in terms of what we believe (take to be true). If that is the case, we would have to prefer the second argument over the first. But, clearly, we can see the former is reasonable while the latter is not. So as an empirical hypothesis that interpretation (explanation in terms of belief) is inescapable, here is the counterexample that shows this claim to be false. That people believe in interpretation is a choice: it's not a fact.

In the rare case that a deductive argument is valid *and* the premises are true, the argument is called *sound*. Here is an example of a sound deductive argument:

Premise 1: Ethics is a subfield of Philosophy.
Premise 2: Philosophy employs logic to derive conclusions from theories.
Conclusion: Ethics employs logic to derive conclusions from theories.

These examples show that focusing on inferential support as in a logically valid argument, and the truth of the propositions in question, are orthogonal matters. We cannot focus on both at once as they lead us in different directions. Hence, in order to get to the conclusion that an argument is sound (both valid and comprised of true propositions) we need to first determine its validity. If it is valid, we can then check if the reasons and conclusion are true. If they are, the argument is sound. But if we mistakenly believe that the truth is the most important aspect of an argument, then we end up endorsing nonsense as though it is logic. Hence, as Patañjali teaches in the *Yoga Sūtra*, we have to disrupt the harm (of interpretation first), and then we can worry about the truth (YS II.30–35).

A second important form of reason is called *induction*. Inductive arguments are used in polling and meteorology, for instance. They also show up in science, for example in epidemiology. Inductive arguments start with a pool of data, and the conclusion of such arguments is a generalization. When the generalization is supported by the data, the induction is called *strong*. When the data is reliable and the conclusion is supported by the data, the induction is called *cogent*. When the generalization is not supported by the data, it is called *weak*. Unlike deductive arguments, the merit of an inductive argument has to do with the conclusion going beyond the evidence. Hence, inductive arguments help us draw big-picture conclusions on the basis of a much narrower set of considerations. Unlike deductive arguments, they are *ampliative*. As in the case of deductive arguments, bad inductive arguments can be comprised of reliable data and true conclusions. What they are missing is the logical connection.

For instance, imagine a pollster who collected information from polling, and the populations that were polled represented the larger population from which they were drawn. But instead of formulating a generalization on the basis of that poll, the pollster tacked on a perfectly true but irrelevant generalization about the weather. This would be a case where the data was reliable and the conclusion true, but the induction was weak.

Or imagine a pollster who conducted interviews but on a sample of voters that was insufficiently sized or not representative of the electorate. If she were to draw any generalization on the basis of that polling, she would have a *strong* induction. It would not, however, be cogent. But if she were to correct the sample so that it represented the larger population that it was drawn from, then any generalization based on that appropriate sample would be a *cogent* induction.

The third and important variety of logic is called *inference to the best explanation* (IBE) or sometimes *abduction*. This is a form of reasoning that occurs frequently in science. Whenever we want to explain something and we have competing theories to choose from, and we make a case that one of the explanations is the best, we are engaging in IBE. For instance, when scientists were made aware of a new illness in 2019, they had several options. They could explain it as just another flu. They could explain it as a bacterial infection. Or they could search for a new explanation. The established theory is that the new illness that appeared in 2019 was a result of a previously unknown virus: SARS-CoV-2. In the case of science, there are criteria that scientists consider in adjudicating between competing theories. Certainly, predictive success is an important factor in selecting the best theory. Unlike inductive arguments, abductive arguments are not ampliative. But like inductive arguments they are not measured by way of the deductive criterion of validity. Rather, abductive arguments turn on success criteria (often discipline relative) that help us select a winning explanation

Irrational people get confused about the relationship between truth and reason. The irrational person, in confusing truth and reason, believes falsely that something reasonable has to conform to what is true. But as we have seen, truth and reason diverge. In the case of IBE, when scientists select the *best* theory to explain a phenomenon, it is the best, *relative to the known options.* It is wholly consistent with such reasoning that a better theory might come along or that the information that needs to be explained is augmented due to new findings. Because reasoning is not the same as what is true, or what we believe is true, it allows us to be dynamic in the face of new data and new challenges.

All three kinds of logic play an important role in breaking the grip that a *saṃskāra* has on us. In Chapter 2, we explored this topic and observed that '*saṃskāra*' is the *Yoga Sūtra* word for an interpretive practice. A *saṃskāra* grips us because of our attachment to the explanation and because it creates a reality on the basis of the interpretive expectations it employs to interpret. If I carry around the belief that I am scared of dogs, and then I use this belief to structure my relating to actual dogs, my fear of dogs is a deductive entailment of my belief. But I will also create an inductive generalization of my being scared of dogs, *all the time.* And it will seem to me that the best explanation for this is either that dogs are scary or I'm a person who is definitively scared of dogs. But logic has been corrupted in these cases. Actual logic is not stuck on any particular belief; it is free to consider a wide assortment of data and explanations. What this brings to light is the ways in which I have convinced myself of something (of being scared of dogs) when there is *no independent evidence* for this. When we reason, we can consider *all sorts of independent evidence.* For instance, I can take in data about dogs in general and their relationships to humans. On the basis of this, I could arrive at a cogent induction. I would learn that on the whole dogs and humans have such a good relationship that in general there is little reason to be frightened about dogs. When we interpret and employ a *saṃskāra*, we are basically corrupting logic from something that allows us to organize and consider various options and then appreciate and experience our own independence into something that recreates self-fulfilling prophecies.

This appreciation of the way logic helps us get over *saṃskāra*-s explains how Yoga, as an activity invested in logical thinking, helps us get over *saṃskāra*-s. When we operate according to *saṃskāra*-s, we live a reactive life. This feels safe, but it actually undermines our opportunities to be an agent. Agency isn't reactivity. It involves deliberation and choice, which are important and basic parts of Yoga as a practice.

Further, the American Psychiatric Association's *Diagnostic and Statistical Manual of Mental Disorders, Fifth Edition (DSM-5)*, in its chapter 'Personality Disorders', describes Narcissistic Personality Disorder as an inflated sense of self and a need for this inflated sense to be acknowledged by others, without any concern for them. Interpretation is the methodology of narcissism: in elevating one's own beliefs to the standard of explanation, one is grandiosely elevating one's own perspective, treating it as though it deserves admiration, but also engaging in a procedure that makes it impossible to understand others who do not share one's perspective, thereby rendering empathy impossible. Adopting a life of *saṃskāra*-s, and thereby interpretation as a methodology, is a methodological foundation for narcissism.

And so the *Yoga Sūtra* begins with a contrast between two approaches to the data (YS I.2–4). On the one hand, we can take responsibility for organizing and understanding what follows from various possibilities we can contemplate, allowing us to maintain our independence as people from what we are contemplating. This is what we do when we engage in logic-based practices. *Or* we allow ourselves to be influenced by what we contemplate, as in the case of a *saṃskāra*. For Yoga, there's only one clear option: the anti-Yoga option is narcissistic but, importantly, irrational and it fails to respect our autonomy. In Yoga, the *ethical and the logical* come to the same thing. There is no way to be a reasonable person while engaging in the selfishness of interpretation. And hence, when we come to examine what the *Yoga Sūtra* says about the end of Yogic practice, it has to do with abandoning the narcissism of interpretation (YS IV.29–34).

Going forward, the most important feature of Yoga to keep in mind is that it is objective, like logic. In the Western tradition, objectivity is often confused with truth. As everyone has a different view of what is true, it seems like objectivity is just a subjective idea, dependent upon your point of view. But objectivity is not the same as truth. It is rather what we can converge on *as we* disagree. When we view a table in a room from differing angles, it appears different to us owing to what aspect of it we view, but nevertheless it's the same table that we are viewing, and the table's various sides explains the differences in our observations. This is why the table is objective. Logic is objective as it is not reducible to truth or what we believe. It is objective in so far as we can converge on the validity of a deductive argument (for instance) or its failure to be valid *independently* of our subjective opinions on whether the premises and conclusions of the argument are true. Yoga as an exercise that helps us embrace logic as a means of sorting the data is hence an exercise in objectivity. Just like logic, it requires that we put on hold our opinions and perspective and consider what we could disagree about. This is an important theme of Yoga – and logic, which we will revisit.

To recap, when trying to interact with and understand the data, we have two options. On the one hand, we could use logic to understand and organize the data. In the case of understanding Philosophy *and other people*, we would use explication. To explicate is to use logical validity (the criterion of good deductive arguments) to deduce a *theory* from a perspective that logically entails its various controversial claims. So if we were explicating South Asian discussions of dharma, we would look to each perspective to render explicit, via logical validity, its theory of dharma. Then we understand the concept of *DHARMA* as what competing theories of dharma disagree about. I was the first to do this (sadly no one had done it before). What this shows is that the disagreement is about *THE RIGHT OR THE GOOD*, *and* Yoga is a fourth basic ethical theory. *Or* we could interpret. This is ordinary. When we interpret, we use our beliefs to understand others. That's to engage in methodological narcissism. That's unfortunately ordinary and prominently employed in the academic literature.

FOUR BASIC THEORIES

While logic is something taught by philosophers to students in university *all the time*, the study of South Asian philosophy has been largely taken over by people without any interest in philosophy. So it is not surprising that no one had bothered to use logic to understand the options from the South Asian tradition and that it was routinely interpreted instead. When we consider how interpretation is itself an outcome of the West's basic theory of thought – the *Linguistic Account of Thought* – this shift away from logic and toward beliefs as the basis of explaining South Asian philosophy is an unsurprising outcome of Western colonialism. We do not have to follow that mistaken route. If we do, we *interpret*: explain everything in terms of our beliefs. If we reject this, we can *explicate*. To explicate is to first use logical validity to render *explicit* a theory that logically entails its controversial claims about a topic, like dharma, and then we can deduce that the concept *DHARMA* is what the competing theories of dharma are disagreeing about. And if we were to engage in this explicatory activity, we would observe that these competing theories are disagreeing about *THE RIGHT OR THE GOOD*. The right pertains to choice and activity, while the good pertains to outcome and accomplishment. *THE RIGHT OR THE GOOD* is also the concept we would discover if we explicated Western ethical theories: we would appreciate that the three ethical theories that Prof. Chidi Anagonye refers to are in fact dissenting theories about this same concept. But when we actually bother to spell this out, we observe that the list of the three major ethical theories in the Western tradition is incomplete and there is space for a fourth basic ethical theory, which is Yoga. And whereas the usual myth is that for ethical reflection we can't find anything sophisticated in South Asia, but it can be found in the West, South Asia has a wider, more complete spread of basic ethical theories that are explored. The famous and perhaps most ancient option from the *Western* tradition is:

- Virtue Ethics: The Good (character, constitution) conditions or produces the Right (choice, action).

In the Western tradition, this theory goes back to Plato and Aristotle. In the South Asian tradition, the most salient Virtue Ethicists are the Jains. Plato and Aristotle – and Confucius in the Chinese tradition – thought that virtue is unevenly distributed. Some people are born lacking the virtues. Others have the raw ability that needs to be cultivated. Those who lack the virtues would be lucky to find someone who has them and will tell them what to do. Theism is a version of Virtue Ethics. It claims that God is the ultimately good moral agent, and hence what God wants is what we should all do. There are many South Asian examples. The ancient Jains hold that an essential trait of every living being (*jīva*) is virtue (*vīrya*). And while we ought to live in accordance with this, ordinarily we get confused with our activity and this causes us to live bad lives that are harmful. Returning to our intrinsic virtue leads to a life that harms no other being and liberates us from our own suffering. Nonaction is on the Jain account superior to action. It is the active choice of *ahiṃsā* (not hurting things) in conformity to our intrinsic virtue.

- Consequentialism: The Good (end) justifies the Right (choice, action).

There are different forms of Consequentialism. The famous form, Utilitarianism, claims that good things we should aim for are not particular to individuals but something we share, like happiness. On a Utilitarian account, we ought to do things that increase happiness, and we ought to do things that minimize displeasure, sadness, and unhappiness.

In the Western tradition, Consequentialism is associated with Jeremy Bentham and John Stuart Mill, though elements of it can be found in Plato and Aristotle. John Stuart Mill was a colonizer of South Asia and also typically Western. He thought that people should be free to experiment to determine what makes them happy but that South Asians were not mature enough for this freedom (*On Liberty* ch. 1). Ironically, his theory is an alteration of Yoga, which he appropriated from South Asia. He also held (in his *Utilitarianism*) that human happiness was more important than nonhuman pleasure: better Socrates dissatisfied than a pig satisfied. Mill's teacher Jeremy Bentham was unusual in the Western tradition. He argued that discriminating against beings on the basis of their species is wrong. What really matters, he argues in his *Principles of Morals and Legislation*, is whether a being can suffer or not. We ought to choose in ways that minimize suffering for all concerned. In South Asia, this is the position that we find in Buddhist Dharma. According to ancient Buddhism, the end we should be minimizing is discomfort (*dukkha*). Buddhist practice is hence justified in so far as it minimizes suffering.

- Deontology: The Right (procedure) justifies the Good (actions, called duties, or omissions, called rights).

In the Western tradition, Kant is the most famous of Deontologists. Like all Deontologists, Kant holds that there are many good things to do, but only some of them are obligatory. The good things to do that are obligatory are selected by some procedure of choosing and doing. Kant's procedure for choosing what is obligatory is called the *Categorical Imperative*, which he elaborates in his *Groundwork of the Metaphysics of Morals*. The main idea behind the Categorical Imperative is that it is a way of choosing that *obliges* everything in the categories of humans/persons. Kant unfortunately is not very clear about this. He has *four* different formulations of the Categorical Imperative, and it's not clear that they all lead to the same conclusions. In the South Asian tradition, the salient example of Deontology is *Karma Yoga* in the *Bhagavad Gītā*. We shall examine this in detail when we dive into the *Gītā* in Chapter 6. In short, Kṛṣṇa recommends that we identify the activities that define our social relationships with others and perfect those activities. So if I am a father and professor, I ought to work on perfecting those activities as a way to relate to myself and others. And this applies *even if* I'm better at doing something else (such as bowling or going for a swim). Better one's own dharma poorly performed than another's well performed (*Gītā* 3.35).

These three ethical theories that are popular in the Western tradition and the South Asian tradition have one thing in common: they provide an account of what we should be doing in terms of practical success (the good). The fourth ethical theory, unheard of in the West, is unique as it does not define what we should choose or do in terms of the good.

- Bhakti/Yoga: The Right (devotion to the procedural ideal, Īśvara) conditions or produces the Good.

Yoga/Bhakti is the opposite of Virtue Ethics. Virtue Ethics claims that one begins with a successful character and it is from this success that right choice and doing follows. Yoga/Bhakti, in contrast, claims that we have to begin with working on the right choosing and doing by being devoted to (*bhakti*) the ideal of right choosing and doing: Īśvara. Success is just the perfection of this practice of devotion. This success is brought about by practising the essential traits of this ideal of the Right, which amounts to doing the right thing. These essential traits that are the component practices of the devotion to the right are unconservative self-challenge (*tapas*) and ownership, self-determination and responsibility to the values we set ourselves (*svādhyāya*) (YS II.1).

Yoga/Bhakti is often confused with Theism (indeed, I've made this mistake in my own writing). Īśvara, to whom the Yogi is devoted, seems like God. But Theism is a version of Virtue Ethics, and Yoga is the opposite. The main difference between Īśvara and typical ideas of theistic God is that the theist's God is already successful: already and essentially Good. Īśvara, in contrast, is the work and practice one has to perfect to be good. Īśvara hence is not Good: it is Right.

Yoga/Bhakti described as a position on the relationship of THE RIGHT OR THE GOOD is a normative ethical theory. Yoga/Bhakti is also what is called a *metaethical* position, a position that helps us understand what is involved in ethical inquiry and discourse. This is Yoga as a responsible approach to understanding the data, which helps us organize thinking and the data into explicated content (YS I.2–3). By engaging in a responsible ordering of the data and thinking, we are also exemplifying what is involved in Yoga as an activity of Devotion to Sovereignty. We are challenging ourselves to depart from past prejudices and beliefs to contemplate thoughts we may not agree with (*tapas*), while also reserving our own right to determine our own choices (*svādhyāya*).

HISTORY, EXPLICATION, AND *W*AC-KY 'YOGA'

An interesting implication of Yoga, this basic ethical theory, is that it is possible for us to genuinely practise Yoga, while subscribing to ideals that are not explicitly part of the central theory. That's the whole point of *svādhyāya*: self-governance. Hence, while one cannot be a Theist, that is a Virtue Ethicist, who genuinely practises Yoga, as part of one's devotion to Īśvara – the practice of being responsible for one's choices – one could transparently choose the values or teachings of Jesus or Muhammad *as a personal choice* as opposed to a choice about what is true for everyone. So in this limited sense Christian or Muslim Yoga is possible. But there is a catch. To actually be practising Yoga, and not an alternative ethical theory, like Virtue Ethics (and its 'religious' version, Theism), one's deference to such values has to be part of one's own practice of *taking back* one's independence by a full devotion to Īśvara. That means that in addition to the self-governing choice, one must also be practising unconservatism, and as noted, a solidarity with people defined by their interest in Sovereignty. This marriage of the unconservatism and self-governance of Yoga is a self-critical journey that may involve critically disavowing some teachings associated with, say, Jesus or Muhammad. Most crucially, within the practice of Yoga, these figures are not venerated because they are in a position to tell us what to do, but because we choose them as our example. It is our power to give when we treat them as our examples, and our power to take back when we choose not to. And in exercising this power, we freely accept the power of others to do the same.

South Asian dharma philosophy, and Yoga as a basic ethical theory, is a threat to *W*estern colonialism in two ways. First, it undermines the idea that the *W*est provides us with all the options to choose from. The very reality of there being a rich history of dharma philosophy in South Asia shows this is false. But this rich history also contains within it an ethical theory that is unheard of in the *W*estern tradition. This ethical theory, Yoga, is anticolonial. Colonialism attempts to impose a perspective on us. Yoga is about getting rid of perspective as a means of understanding, and placing our energy into right choosing and doing. The activity of being devoted to the ideal of Right choosing and doing, Īśvara, is Devotion to Sovereignty. Colonialism as an attempt to impede people's independence is *anti-yogic*, as it violates and ignores the essential value of Yoga.

Yoga as an anticolonial moral and political philosophy was developed as a response to a concern about the possibilities of being free. The ancient tradition in the *W*est began with a different batch of constraints.

In the last chapter, we observed how LAT encouraged and supported the ancient *W*estern commitment to communitarianism: the idea that the individual is defined by, or only understands their role in, community. This was a straightforward outcome of the presumed LAT. But so too is anthropocentrism – the idea that when we are thinking about dharmic questions, we are restricted to humans (nonhumans do not count). This is because ethics in this tradition is about community membership based on the same (human) language and reasons: *logos*.

Ancient South Asia: Vedas, Sāṅkhya, Jainism, and Buddhism

Ancient South Asians were free to abandon anthropocentric and communitarian modes of understanding because language was not foundational. The Vedas (beginning 1500 BCE) teach us that as animals we live in a world of natural forces (*devas*) that exert pressures on us, which we must feed to avoid bad things. Given their power over us, we must sacrifice to please these natural forces. If nothing else, we must appropriate the bodies of other living beings to feed our metabolic fire (*Aitareya Āraṇyaka* I.1.2). The ancient Vedic peoples saw this arrangement as unfair and necessary (*Aitareya Brāhmana* 2.1.7). But given their interest in the ends of avoiding disease and living successfully, they treated these sacrifices as justified by the ends. They were in effect Consequentialists. Importantly, their ethical outlook was what Nietzsche later called resentful: the goods of life (like health) are understood in terms of avoiding the bads (like disease, starvation, and death). This is resentful because it prevents trusting and enjoying life without distrusting its bads. As the South Asian philosophical tradition grows, questions of dharma, or ethics, are posed against the backdrop of the apparent determinacy of the universe versus the needs and requirements of responsible individuals. Responsibility requires free will. External causes limit our freedom.

With the advent of systematic philosophy, this picture of the universe as an evolution of cosmic natural forces that exert pressures on individuals who are patients of its processes is codified in the philosophy of Sāṅkhya as found in Īśvarakṛṣṇa's *Sāṅkhya Kārikā* (200 CE). According to this theory, history is the evolution of nature (*prakṛti*) from simpler to more complex states with emergent properties like senses, mind, and intellect. We have to acknowledge the reality of a diversity of people, on this account, as nature is the same for us all, but our perspectives are unique. The individual understanding the difference between people and nature frees us from this forced experience. But this understanding itself is something facilitated by nature: it gives us this experience, and in the final analysis, it was nature that went through various states of existence. We just watched it happen as though it was us living and doing things (SK 62).

Sāṅkhya paints a tragic picture. Our experiences are real and uncontrollable because we are external observers of natural-order events that we cannot influence. Ancient Buddhist Consequentialism modifies this picture. According to the early *Mahānidānasutta* and in later works like Nāgārjuna's *Mūlamadhyamakakārikā*, ancient Buddhism (circa 500 BCE) views reality as conditioned and caused by natural factors. This is the principle of *dependent origination*. Whereas on a Sāṅkhya account, people are external observers of causal relations (what it calls *prakṛti*), on the Buddhist account, there is nothing external to the relationships of causes and events. Hence observers, people, are really special, psychologically loaded aspects of dependent origination. By deconstructing the idea of our estrangement from reality, Buddhism argues that we can choose to reduce difficult experiences because we are not external observers of our experiences. Our ordinary idea of individuality is the cause of problems, and this individuality is tied to a subjective variety of motivation that is out of step with objectivity: desire. This is explained in the Four Noble Truths, as found in the *Dhammacakkappavattana Sutta* (*Saṃyutta Nikāya* 56.II).

The First Truth is that, ordinarily, life is difficult ('*dukkha*' in Pāli). The Second Truth is that there is a cause of this suffering: desire (in Pāli '*taṇhā*'). Desire as a motivation is problematic as it is an agent-relative (and agent-particular) motivation. But this is subjective, and the objectivity of reality (as a continuity of causes) does not support this kind of subjectivity, and hence it causes suffering. The Third Truth is that there is an end to this problem. And the Fourth Truth is the truth about the path that gets rid of this suffering. This is often formalized as the Eightfold Path:

1. Right View (*Sammā Diṭṭhi*)
2. Right Intention (*Sammā Sankappa*)
3. Right Speech (*Sammā Vācā*)
4. Right Action (*Sammā Kammanta*)
5. Right Livelihood (*Sammā Ājīva*)
6. Right Effort (*Sammā Vāyāma*)
7. Right Mindfulness (*Sammā Sati*)
8. Right Conclusion (*Sammā Samādhi*).

Noteworthy is that this is a *path* or a *way to an end*: this is a Consequentialist model. (For those interested in comparing this Eightfold Path with the Eight Limbs of Yoga, which we will study in the next two chapters, the metaphor of 'limbs' in Yoga is about *implementation*, which is a procedural notion. In Yoga, we go nowhere.)

Another alternative or amendment to the Sāṅkhya picture is the Jain Virtue Ethical amendment. Jainism (500 BCE) divides reality into natural or material, on the one hand, and a diversity of distinct living beings (*jīva*-s) or selves, on the other. This aspect resembles the Sāṅkhya picture. However, Jains view the association of selves and nature as voluntary but also a confusion. When selves attempt to act, they traverse their own boundaries and make choices that constitute an enmeshment with the natural world. This always results in harm for the agent and other living beings. This is because action (karma) is not in keeping with our intrinsic virtue (*vīrya*), which transcends activity. While we can act, we should strive for nonaction, and this allows us to disentangle ourselves from the natural world and live a life of freedom.[1]

Cosmic Colonialism and the Yoga Response

Vedic ethics evolve beyond naturalism and resentment. By 700 BCE, the *Upaniṣads* had shifted focus. The *Upaniṣads* view the self as ultimately responsible for its life and understand it as a procedural substance of Brahman: growth, expansion, development. The earlier tradition focused on external causation. So whereas the earlier Vedas explained the self as being on the receiving end of natural forces and pressures, the later Vedas reunderstand the self as existing with a substance of growth and expansion. What that means is that life experiences and challenges are to be reunderstood not as a matter of external pressure but an internal pressure to grow. Here, the self is given a bigger role in accounting for life experiences. Moreover, in time, the distinction between the earlier nature-based practice (*prakṛti*) and the latter emphasis on the self (*puruṣa*) becomes two contrasting approaches to life that Yoga begins with. And like the Vedic tradition, the argument is in favour of moving toward the self as the centre of life.

The *Upaniṣads* now explain Yoga as an option. We shall look at the famous dialogue in the *Upaniṣads* in which the god Death explains Yoga to the boy Nāciketa who faces Death ahead of time in Chapter 6. In short, we can note that Yoga is classically explained here as the responsible ordering of mind, body, sense, and intellect to protect individual autonomy. Its opposite, conflation of the self with objects of awareness, leads to personal ruin (*Kaṭha Upaniṣad* I.3).

If we want to understand the origins of the anticolonialism of Yoga, we need to go back to its start. For what Yoga grows out of is a concern for *cosmic colonialism*. Colonialism is having a perspective thrust upon us as something we have to accommodate and live in accordance with. It succeeds when this perspective is internalized as part of the colonized way of life. Cosmic colonialism is the perspective(s) of the gods, natural forces, which are forcing themselves on us, because in reality they are part of a system that exudes and passes along pressure and coercion. Sāṅkhya normalizes this: that's just the way things are, and we are in effect fooled into thinking we have some independent agency. Jainism claims that's the way it is, and we need to get ourselves out of this mess by not participating in it at all. Buddhism claims that cosmic colonialism is really only a problem when we act subjectively as though we are exceptions to these dependently originating pressures. We need to rather abandon our individuality and accept that we aren't anything but aspects of the system. Then we can choose in a way that minimizes the coercive aspects of the system of dependently originating phenomena. Yoga, in contrast, opts to resist cosmic colonialism by denying that it is the only way to organize ourselves. Participating in it is a choice, and there is an alternative:

Yogic resistance. Yogic resistance is possible because there is an alternative to the natural approach to life, which consists in buying our experiences of the system as our own identity. And that is to adopt a life of choice and responsibility to ensure that all aspects of our life respect our intrinsic interest in independence. This is a practice of ever-continuous activism. Western colonialism, White Supremacy, and any other example of systemic oppression is just another version of cosmic colonialism on a Yoga account. It seems to those who can participate in this project of colonialism that everything is going their way. But really, they have lost their independence to a system of oppression. Overcoming colonialism is hence not about denying it as a possibility but doing something else with your energy and time: Yoga – *Īśvara praṇidhāna*.

These reflections show that Yoga is *not* the same as Sāṅkhya. It is not even a version of Sāṅkhya. When we explicate the options, we see that Sāṅkhya is the view that nature is the primary explanation of life, and the self, or person, is nothing but a spectator. It is from Sāṅkhya that we get the idea that the self is pure consciousness. Yoga, in contrast, is a *second order* philosophy that contrasts two competing methodologies: the yogic method of persons (*puruṣa*), explication, consists of being responsible for our relationship to mental content by way of responsibility for everything else (such as our sense and intellect) to maintain our own independence, in contrast to anti-Yoga, which consists in interpretation. This second method is the method of nature (*prakṛti*): of external influence. Whereas according to Sāṅkhya, persons have no power and are not agents but mere spectators, Yoga makes choice, responsibility, and activity primary to the self. The Yoga self is the self that is responsible for its life.

In emphasizing responsibility, the Yogic picture of the self is very similar to the *Upaniṣad* view of the self as something that is the account of its life, seated in the substance of growth and expansion. But the standard *Upaniṣad* views simply emphasize the self and do not emphasize the methodological choice before us, so there is a divergence there between what is standardly taught in the *Upaniṣads* and Yoga.

Vedānta, Monism, and Western Colonialism

Another important point of departure is the school called Vedānta. 'Vedānta' literally means 'end of Vedas': it is hence the position we learn about in the *Upaniṣads*. The *Upaniṣads* say all sorts of things. They are not consistent.

Some *Upaniṣads* talk about the self as though there is only one universal Self indistinguishable from Brahman. Others talk about a diversity of selves. Owing to this ambiguity, and the fact that it was thought to be rude to claim to have an original idea in the South Asian tradition, there was a *Sūtra* that tried to summarize the view in the *Upaniṣads*, called the *Vedānta Sūtra* (or *the Brahma Sūtra*), and then numerous commentaries on this summary, with very different views. Rāmānuja (1017–1137 CE), perhaps the most influential of commentators on the *Vedānta Sūtra*, tried to reconcile the various views of the self in the Vedas via a Yogic twist. He argued that while indeed there is a universal Self – Īśvara – which is the same as Viṣṇu (*tapas*) and Lakṣmī (*svādhyāya*), there are numerous individual selves that are bodily expressions of this highest Self. Bhakti (what Patañjali calls Yoga) is essential to liberating ourselves from difficulty, and this devotion allows us to align our activity with our shared, higher, universal Self: Īśvara. The position defended by Rāmānuja is in a large way basically what we find in the *Yoga Sūtra*, though this is not usually appreciated – even by Rāmānuja who often claims to be articulating a different view (*Śrī Bhāṣya* 2.1.3). Then, there is another earlier commentator who is probably better known outside of India: Śaṅkara. Śaṅkara's position is very much like what we find in the *Sāṅkhya Kārikā*, but with a twist. According to Śaṅkara (circa 750 CE), our individual picture of ourselves is an illusion constructed out of nature (*prakṛti*) that gives us the experience of choosing and doing. But really, there is only a bare, universal Self (which is basically pure consciousness) and when we get over the illusion of the individual self, constructed out of nature, we are free (Śaṅkara's *Brahma Sūtra Bhāṣya*, preamble). This is called 'Advaita' or 'No-Second' Vedānta. In English we call this kind of position Monistic – it only acknowledges one thing: the universal Self.

There are many more versions of Vedānta. Another radically different position (which appears to be a result of Western influence) is defended by Madhva (1238–1317 CE). According to Madhva, everything is unique and different, and each one of us is defined by our character. Some are eternally liberated, others are eternally damned because they are essential vicious, and the rest of us transmigrate in a purgatory forever – a position much like what is defended in Plato's *Phaedrus*. Then there's the Difference-and-non-different (Bhedhābedha) view that is famously associated with ISKCON (the Hare Kṛṣṇa movement) that holds that we are all the same as, but also different from, the ultimate Self.

The idea that there is *one* position called Vedānta is a misrepresentation or an outright lie. One origin of this misinformation is partisan schools of Vedānta education, based on Advaita teaching. While Advaita Vedānta is always just one position among many in South Asia, Western colonialism ironically made it very popular. During colonialism, many South Asian intellectuals who were deeply wounded by colonial criticisms of South Asia chose to show that South Asians can do what the colonizer does but better. At the time, British Idealism of Bradley, based on the thought of Hegel - a version of Monism - was popular in the West, and many South Asians chose to champion this as though it were the only form of Vedānta. Given that Monism was already popular in the West, Advaita Vedānta was well received by Westerners. South Asians who internalized Western colonialism started to champion Monism as the only or basic option of South Asia.

Monism is actually an ancient position that goes back to Plato himself. On the basis of Plato's teachings, which identified the Good as the highest reality and everything as a derivation of this Good (see the *Republic* 509d–511e), *Platonists* such as Plotinus called the Good the One, which emanates a kind of light that becomes dimmer as it travels from the core. The further these emanations travel, the more experiential they become until they end up being material, which according to Plotinus is *evil* (*Ennead* I.8). Matter is evil because it is the furthest from the Goodness of the One. In other words, the physical world is not reformable by our activity owing to its very nature as furthest from the Good. There can be no point to activism or social progress as that's basically impossible in this physical world. Later on, the racist and White Supremacist Albert Schweitzer wrote a very influential book called *Indian Thought and Its Development* (1936), which claimed that Indian thought was world and life negating, turning its back on the ethical challenges of life, while ethics presumes life affirmation. This is actually Plotinus's view. This projection of Plotinus on to South Asia is to be echoed in the equally racist Indologists who either explicitly denied the reality of South Asian moral philosophy or upheld Schweitzer's White Supremacy by simply not talking about Indian moral philosophy. And this is, of course, an essential core of Western colonialism: it has to depict the European tradition as a practical saviour and BIPOC traditions as lacking any practical wisdom - namely, moral (dharma) philosophy. Academic Indology with its notable absence of any serious and professionally appropriate discussion of South Asian moral philosophy is an important part of the project of Western colonialism. It's not just a lacuna. It's an intentional incompetence that arises from intentionally engaging in *W*estern interpretation. If you think Schweitzer's 1936 book was published a long time ago and things have changed: they haven't. The *W*estern scholarship on South Asia, especially by self-appointed Indologists, has not examined the rich history of South Asian moral philosophy, for that would involve getting rid of the *W*AC-ky foundations of Indology.

In reality, in the Yoga tradition, the Earth is a goddess, Bhūmi, a version of the goddess of *svādhyāya* (self-governance), Lakṣmī. She is also materiality and material wealth. The world is to be celebrated and valued in the South Asian tradition. Schweitzer's racist position, a projection of the Platonist beginnings of the *W*estern tradition, is confused. But it is true that Advaita Vedānta of Śaṅkara, out of the many options that are called 'Vedānta', converges with Platonism in criticizing worldly possibilities: Plato also famously entertained the idea of transmigration (we find this affirmed in Advaita Vedānta too). Moreover, while the ethical life on Śaṅkara's account is part of an ordinary confused life based on the natural illusion of individuality, an enlightened approximation of universal oneness leads us to appreciate that dharma is an evil for those who want to be free (Śaṅkara *Gītā Bhāṣya* 4.21, see also 2.11). This entails a futility of ethical activity in the world, which overlaps with Plotinus's assessment.

So when *W*esterners love Vedānta, and by that they mean Advaita Vedānta, it has a lot to do with *W*estern *saṃskāra*-s and *W*AC-ky approaches to South Asia. By no means is this evidence of learning about South Asian philosophy, for it involves ignoring the diversity of options that are Vedānta and conflating it with Advaita. And often this love of Advaita Vedānta happens in circles where people claim to be interested in Yoga, which is distinct. This unfortunately defines a generation of *W*estern appropriation of South Asian philosophy. And to what political end? Well, if we're all one, there is no grounds for criticizing anyone for doing anything other than what one is doing. And as the world is deeply problematic owing to being so far removed from the source, there's no way for us to engage in any type of political criticism of colonialism. What you see, on this view, is as good as it gets, which, by the way, is bad.

YOGA ETHICS FOR TEACHING AND PRACTICE

I was guest teacher at a large online 300-hour YTT. During my talk, I told the group that the most absurd thing I hear about is the idea of yoga 'off the mat'

– as though Yoga is primarily something you do on a mat. I exclaimed: there's no mat in any ancient philosophy about Yoga. The entire reduction of yoga to something that is on a mat is a fabrication. Really, Yoga is fundamentally a moral and political exercise of creating space for ourselves as autonomous people. At this moment, one of the facilitators – a racialized woman – got upset and interjected. She rebuked me for making such a claim. She continued to inform me and everyone present that yoga on a mat in a class is one of the few times that people such as her get to take a break from the stress of the day. It is a sacred space where she gets to put aside moral and political issues and simply focus on her breath and posture. In effect, I was insensitive for trying to erase this ritualized space of amorality and apolitical activity. My response was two-fold.

First, to decide that we need a break from the moral and political activism of Yoga is like deciding that we need a break from standing up for ourselves and protecting our interest in independence. If we act like that in yoga spaces, we act as though people's boundaries are not relevant to the practice of yoga. And then yoga practice becomes a space for abuse. Rather, yoga teachers really have a responsibility for making sure that spaces where people teach and practise yoga are also cared for by way of yoga ethics and politics. This ensures that people can practise successfully without moral or political harm.

Second, and more importantly, when we *really* practise Yoga, we simplify our life. Everywhere we go and everything we do, it's always the same practice. Before I was a Yogi, I had different versions of myself that I trotted out depending upon the context. Now, it's always the same me showing up everywhere with the same devotional practice, where I work on my own unconservatism and self-governance while I ensure that the space I'm in is safe for people to own their own autonomy. This practice has no pause or break. I'm like this with my family, with my colleagues, with my neighbours, and when I go grocery shopping. I don't have to worry about how I'm going to negotiate my various social interactions, for it's always the same devotional practice that facilitates my interaction with others.

As I continued to teach, she slowly started to calm down. To my surprise, she started to follow me on Instagram. For me this was more evidence that being intense and ever committed to Yoga allows everyone else to find themselves among a flurry of pain and emotions.

But the event also showed me how (some) YTTs clearly do not set students up to deal with the ethics of yoga teaching with any success. This yoga teacher in charge of teaching yoga teachers should have known better. YTTs wouldn't have to worry about teaching about ethics if they simply taught Yoga. For then, what students would be learning is the moral and political activism of Yoga, which would furnish them with *all* of the checks and balances needed to teach responsibly. As noted in Chapter 2, *WAC*-ky yoga spaces that are characterized by top-down power structures that are hotbeds of abuse and sexual misconduct require a Virtue Ethical paradigm, and Yoga is the very opposite. The reason that Yoga the ethical practice protects each one of us is that in being devoted to Īśvara – Sovereignty – we are devoted to the normative essence of what it is to be a person. And as we act in accordance with this devotion, we create spaces where others can take the opportunity to practise their own devotion to the essence of what it is to be a person. In practising this, we become a model for others to take charge of their own lives and be their own masters. Moral and political abuse, like colonialism, occurs when people are denied the space to be their own masters. Yoga restores this to everyone. It's up to us to practise it. In the next few chapters, we will dive more deeply into what this practice consists of.

CHAPTER 3 REFLECTIONS

» Having been introduced to the idea of ethical theory as a story about the relationship between Right choosing and doing, and Good outcomes, can you identify which ethical theory you subscribe to? Is it the same or different from the one you actually follow?

» If you are serious about yoga, are you serious about Yoga?

» What changes would you have to implement in your life if you were to engage in Yoga as a basic ethical practice? What things would stay the same?

» Is your Yoga education environment clear about the diversity of moral philosophical options in the South Asian tradition – does is it give Yoga the respect it deserves as autonomous option?

» Buddhists and others are Consequentialists: they conceive of dharma as a means to an end. Can you understand how Yoga is not a version of Consequentialism? If not, identify the confusion, and then compare it to

Yoga as the idea that we ought to be devoted to the procedural ideal of personhood: Īśvara.

» Can you list ways in which Yoga brings about benefits as a side effect of practice?

» What is the political point of claiming that we are all one? Do you know people who talk like this? Can you talk about colonialism and racism with them? How could they process the harm done to others that they did not experience?

» What would always practising Yoga (devotion to Īśvara) look like in your life?

» Have you been exposed to Vedānta or Sāṅkhya? Were these clearly explained as distinct options or were they conflated with Yoga?

» How can you use logic in your life to expose your own *saṃskāra*-s? (Hint, examine your assumptions, prejudices, and habits, and assess whether you can understand them as a result of reasoning, or are they based on what you believe is true or is a fact of your life?)

CHAPTER 4

YOGA SŪTRA: ACTIVISM AND SOCIAL JUSTICE (BOOKS 1 AND 2)

INTRODUCTION

Our book is unusual in its anticolonial exploration of Yoga, the philosophy. But as we saw in the previous chapter, Yoga is originally *anticolonial*. So really, our anticolonial focus is simply an explication of Yoga. Exploring the philosophy of Yoga hence requires confronting the colonialism that impacts learning about Yoga. One kind of obvious colonialism is the imposition of a Western perspective on ethical choice on BIPOC, which involves not properly considering and acknowledging the rich history that non-Western traditions have of thinking critically about public life. Yoga is explicitly suppressed in Western colonialism as Yoga is not part of the Western tradition. It is a fourth basic ethical theory, as we saw, that criticizes the narcissistic methodology of colonialism (interpretation) but provides practices to repair the damage of colonialism. We shall consider that in greater detail in this chapter.

While there are a few sources of classical Yoga philosophy, such as the *Upaniṣads* and the *Bhagavad Gītā*, the *Yoga Sūtra* occupies an important place in the articulation of Yoga. The *Yoga Sūtra* is from the period of Indian philosophy (200 BCE–200 CE) when philosophers were composing *sūtra* texts. Sūtra texts are collections of condensed aphorisms that systematically and formally set out a school of thought's position. The word '*sūtra*' can stand both for the whole text and for the individual aphorism. The *Nyāya Sūtra*, for instance, encodes the philosophy of Nyāya. The *Yoga Sūtra* encodes the philosophy of Yoga. Each *sūtra* (aphorism) is like a zip file that has to be decompressed.

This allows dense philosophy to be recorded in a short, memorizable text. The challenge is in the decompression of the text. Diving into the study of this formal period of South Asian philosophy requires philosophical skills to unpack and explicate philosophy that almost all contemporary authors on the topic lack.

This brings us to the nonobvious variety of Western colonialism that is nonetheless a very serious problem: the colonization of the 'academic' literature by Western interpretation. This practice serves to provide intellectual legitimacy to the project of colonialism. And it ultimately serves to *hide* the ethical and social justice dimensions of Yoga.

The current field of commentators in the West, who constitute the major voices of Yoga Studies, are nearly all *not* professional philosophers. It is difficult to observe any BIPOC among them. They are for the most part linguists or ethnographers (students of culture – which encodes language) of European descent. As noted in previous chapters, the West begins with the LAT in the ancient Greek idea of *logos*: one word for thought, and speech. This model of thought confuses thinking with believing, for what we express in language is typically the thoughts we believe. Hence, this tradition, by confusing thinking with believing, is an interpretive tradition, which tries to explain everything in terms of *its* beliefs. But as reasoning is about thinking (appreciating the inferential support that some thoughts provide other thoughts independently of their truth) and believing is really about our attitude that a thought is true, interpretation (explanation in terms of belief) is incompatible with logical thinking as it confuses thoughts with beliefs. Logic is the inferential support thoughts provide for other thoughts. Beliefs are just attitudes: nothing follows from a belief. And yet, thinking, logic, is required to explicate philosophy. So the Western tradition in being grounded in LAT, its most basic *saṃskāra* (interpretive tendency), which undermines reasoning in favour of beliefs expressed in language (a product of culture), produces commentators who adopt Linguistics or an Ethnographic analysis of cultural language practices as the means of study, but for the same reason are unable to reason and understand Philosophy which requires logic. So the problem is not that these authors are linguists or ethnographers. Indeed, I have worked professionally with genuine scholars of South Asia who are originally linguists or ethnographers. What sets (these) scholars apart is that they regard South Asia as something to *learn from*. They do not treat it as something to explain by way of their beliefs. These scholars are already decolonial. In contrast, the

Western tradition, grounded in LAT, makes it seem like Linguistics or an Anthropological analysis of language practices is sufficient for understanding Philosophy written in Sanskrit or expressed contemporarily in modern languages when it is not. *Worse*, LAT, at the foundation of the Western tradition, conflates thinking and believing and thereby *disables* reasoning. In short, the tradition creates logically – philosophically – incompetent linguists and social scientists who mistakenly believe themselves qualified to talk about Yoga (because of their linguistic knowledge) as the loudest voices in the room. What they do instead is they try to interpret everything – and especially South Asia – on the basis of the Western tradition, starting with its most basic *saṃskāra* (interpretive tendency): LAT. Call these writers who operate against the backdrop of the basic *saṃskāra* of the West, Western Indologists or Western Yoga Students. Could one become a professional philosopher and operate according to these same Western principles? Sure. It happens all the time. This is why Philosophy departments in the West are usually happy to leave the study of BIPOC philosophy to non-philosophers or to hire people who lack philosophical training or skill to be their BIPOC Philosophy faculty.

The *Yoga Sūtra* is divided into four books. While the Yoga account of dharma (*THE RIGHT OR THE GOOD*) is the thread that holds the work together, the first two books bring attention to the ethical practice of Yoga. The first book is called the '*Samādhi-pāda*'. '*Samādhi*' is the *Yoga Sūtra* term for conclusion or roundup, but one that reveals the self – the investigator (YS IV.3). The *Samādhi-pāda* hence reviews the items we discover or are aware of to appreciate the practice of Yoga, which reveals ourselves. This includes the basic distinction between the practice of Yoga (explication) and anti-Yoga (interpretation). The second book is the *Sādhana-pāda*. '*Sādhana*' is the *Yoga Sūtra* term for practice. This second book hence not only outlines Yoga as an idealized three-part practice (of *tapas*, *svādhyāya*, and *Īśvara praṇidhāna*), but it also begins an account of Yoga as a *nonideal* political action plan (the Eight Limbs of Yoga). It is the *Yoga Sūtra* that teaches us how to deal with the racism and incompetence that constitutes the barrier to understanding its practical wisdom. But we have to be practising Yoga to unlock this. In the second section of this chapter, we shall focus on the question of how to read the *Yoga Sūtra*. Western colonialism changes what should really be a matter of applying logic-based methods to understanding Yoga and Patañjali into a political exercise of White Supremacy. We shall be clear in identifying its manifestations in the literature and in choosing an alternative approach.

This transparency in how we approach the *Yoga Sūtra* is part of the practice of Yoga. In the third section, we will overview Book 1, the *Samādhi-pāda*, which provides the tools (and more) to confront, expose, and be done with the irrationality of interpretation. In the fourth section, we will review Book 2, the *Sādhana-pāda*. In the last chapter we observed how Buddhism is a different philosophical project from Yoga. In the fifth section we shall conclude this chapter by considering how Yoga is not Stoicism nor WAC-ky Buddhism.

THE LITERATURE (*ĀGAMĀḤ*)

The *W*est, in confusing its beliefs with the facts, complains that activism is a bias that has no place in scholarship. However, engaging in interpretation, which is the methodology of *W*estern colonialism, is all about employing one's bias in explanation. This is ordinary in the 'academic' literature. Activism in response to this is not biased: it is anti-bias. Anticolonial, *activist* research will always be accurate as it involves using logic to tease out implications and thereby circumvent our ego. In Philosophy, this method is explication, which involves rendering explicit what the *Yoga Sūtra* has to teach us via logic. This is always accurate as it does not involve projecting on to the text: rather, it requires rendering explicit reasons and arguments in the text that contribute to a controversy. From the interpretive vantage of *W*estern Indologists or Yoga Students who lack racist beliefs, they will be surprised at the accusation that they are engaging in an exercise of White Supremacy as they evaluate their culpability for racism in terms of their beliefs. As they lack explicitly racist beliefs, they believe themselves to be innocent. But the problem is not reducible to racist beliefs: the racial and racist features of the enterprise are generated by using *W*estern beliefs – especially beliefs in the propriety of interpretation – as the explanation of South Asia. This sets up the *W*estern tradition, the tradition of White people, as the explanation of everything. This is hence literally White Supremacy, and it is normalized in the academic literature. If we look to classical Indian philosophy, no one thought that explanation in terms of what you believe was a good idea. Indeed, what we believe is a function of social conventions that we participate in and constitutes what South Asians called a worldly or conventional variety of truth – *saṃvṛti* or *vyāvahārika satya.* And these conventional truths (like, say, what side of the road to drive on or what counts as an ethical practice among folks we live and interact with) depend upon us believing them to be conventions. So, in

Canada, we drive on the right side of the road. That's a conventional truth. But it's ultimately reducible to our collective belief that the right side of road is the side to drive on. If we Canadians all changed our beliefs on this topic, there would be a different convention to defer to. Similarly, the idea that some things are religions and others are secular is just a convention. The distinction is explained by the beliefs people have about the distinction between the two, and there is a colonial history to this. It turns out that the philosophy of White people is always secular, and if the philosophy has BIPOC roots, it's religious. There is no fact about this model of secularism (what I call Secularism_2 in contrast to Secularism_1 of open philosophical disagreement) apart from shared beliefs about the secular and the religious. This contrasts with ultimate truth – *paramārtha satya*. These are facts that are independent of our beliefs. How we get to them is a matter of debate in the tradition. In Yoga, we arrive at these facts by disrupting the systemic harm of interpretation, by employing Yogic – logical – methodology. We saw in Chapter 3, for instance, that when we employ such methods of explication to South Asia, we do not find religion. We find ethical theory. That's not dependent on our beliefs: if it were, it would be an interpretation. The Western belief that interpretation is the means to understanding BIPOC traditions is reducible to its beliefs and is hence a principal form of White Supremacy.

As Western Indology/Yoga Studies is based on *saṃskāra*-s from the West, it is natural for people who are racialized as White to adopt this approach. Nature in the context of Yoga is the external force of causation: it is what comes to us from the outside. And hence Western *saṃskāra*-s are natural for European descendants as an external force that pressures by way of their ancestral tradition. Unless one adopts an anticolonial practice of resistance, one will adopt ancestral *saṃskāra*-s as their own. When people of European descent adopt these *saṃskāra*-s of the West, they avail themselves of *White privilege*. White privilege is often defined as a series of opportunities and resources available to White people, and not available to others. White people who make use of Western *saṃskāra*-s of interpretation create and foster their own White privilege. Normally, in Western discourse, privilege is treated as a property of the system: so, on this account, White people always have privilege in a world of White Supremacy. But on this Yoga analysis, it's actually a choice to have privilege that comes down to accepting the *saṃskāra*-s of an interpretive tradition. Then we lose our individuality and become agents of the system. Moreover, on a Yoga account, there is no system aside from us internalizing the *saṃskāra*-s that come to us naturally. Any system of oppression, whether one of race, sex, species, or caste, depends upon individuals internalizing that order as though it is their self-interest and then acting to defend it as a matter of self-defence. And we can each do our part to undo the system by abandoning its *saṃskāra*-s. This is to be a Yoga activist, which involves dismantling and disrupting systemic harm to allow for a world of diversity that respects personal boundaries (this is the first limb of Yoga).

When people of European descent employ these *W*estern *saṃskāra*-s to 'study' Yoga, they make themselves the criterion of explaining Yoga. In short, they do not learn: Yoga becomes a prop in the project of *W*AC, which we covered in Chapter 2. So instead of rendering *explicit* what Yoga has to teach us, they tell us about themselves and what they take to be true (what they believe) about Yoga as though that counts as research or scholarship.

A recent example of this is the revealingly titled *The Truth of Yoga* by Daniel Simpson. A work that teaches about Yoga would render explicit its reasons for its conclusions, and this exercise evaluates Yoga in terms of the inferential support its reasons provide for its conclusions. Inferential support is independent from truth. As we saw in Chapter 3, we can focus on either logic or truth but not both. An emphasis on what Simpson takes to be true of Yoga means he is not tracking the reasons of Yoga philosophers. Rather, it tells us more about what Simpson believes is true about Yoga than what Yoga reasons. So the book is really about him. This is typical of the literature. It is written primarily by interpreters who are concerned with sharing their interpretations, and this tells us more about them than what they are writing on.

It is much harder for South Asian and other BIPOC authors to participate in *W*estern Indology and Yoga Studies as it's not part of their ancestral *saṃskāra*-s. BIPOC have to essentially *acquire* a Eurocentric identity and outlook to participate in *W*estern Indology and Yoga Studies and overrun their own Indigenous identity. In acquiring a Eurocentric identity they will help themselves to Eurocentric beliefs that they then use to interpret the South Asian tradition. This is not impossible. For instance, one of the signs of *W*estern Indology is that because it interprets the South Asian tradition from a *W*estern vantage, it simply misses South Asian moral philosophy (that we examined in the previous chapter) and concludes it doesn't exist. Yoga, the fourth basic ethical theory, is hence erased from academic commentary on South Asia. We can hear this acquired *W*estern identity in the voice of the famous and influential South Asian Indologist Bimal Matilal (1989) who claimed that Indian philosophers didn't contribute to moral philosophy because they don't do what 'we' call moral philosophy. The 'we' he includes himself in is a Eurocentric 'we'. If it were a 'we' that included South Asians, he would allow himself to see that South Asians contributed richly to what South Asians call moral (dharma) philosophy.

This toxic, White-Supremacist scene creates pressures that keep BIPOC and South Asian authors from becoming philosophers and writing on South Asian philosophy. Western Indology gate-keeps the peer review of South Asian philosophy in Western publications. There are four signs of this.

First, publications that are supposed to be devoted to the study of South Asian philosophy, like the *Journal of Indian Philosophy*, will simply lack any discussion of explicated South Asian moral philosophy that we are engaging in. This lack of engagement in South Asian moral philosophy defines the field for the simple reason that if we interpret on the basis of the Western tradition, we recreate the colonial presentations of South Asian thought as inherently religious, spiritual, and amoral. If we explicate, we appreciate the colonial illusion of South Asian thought as religious, and rather we see that it was a robust history of moral philosophy. And indeed, to understand the precolonial history, we need to explicate, which virtually no one wants to do. When we explicate, we see that moral philosophy was *the* basic philosophical controversy of the South Asian tradition. When we interpret according to the Western tradition, all moral philosophy from South Asia is wiped away except for some few leftover crumbs.

Second, instead of Philosophy, we find in these places publications on the topic of Linguistics. Examples from the *Journal of Indian Philosophy* include: 'How Many Sounds are in Pāli?',[1] 'The Buddha's Wordplays: The Rhetorical Function and Efficacy of Puns and Etymologizing in the Pali Canon',[2] 'Observations on the Use of Quotations in Sanskrit Dharmanibandhas',[3] and 'Defining the Other: An Intellectual History of Sanskrit Lexicons and Grammars of Persian'.[4]

Third, which is not apparent from the outside: if one sends in academic material to such journals, one is likely to receive 'peer' reviews from non-philosophers who interpret the contribution according to Western *saṃskāra*-s. The irony is that these commentators are not the 'peers' of professional philosophers writing on South Asia. Yet their views are treated as peer review.

Fourth, the colonial trauma of inheriting a colonized understanding of the South Asian tradition (as a religious or spiritual exercise) also ensures that South Asian authors are not equipped to appease the academic gatekeepers who want to assess the tradition in terms of Linguistics while interpreting it according to the *W*estern tradition. Hence, especially in the *W*est, South Asians wanting to study their tradition will find space in Religious Studies but not in Philosophy, which has been taken over and colonized by the non-philosophers of *W*estern Indology. It may not be surprising by now that when I speak to fellow scholars, university professors, and teachers, who are of South Asian descent and work on South Asia, there is near universal agreement that the academic exercise of studying South Asia is racist. We say this to each other in private. In our investigation, we have the explanation for what is observed by South Asian colleagues. The problem is *not* that White people are studying South Asian history and thought. It is that this field is populated by people *interpreting* South Asia on the basis of the *W*estern tradition, and this is much easier for people of European descent for the reasons discussed. And to do so is to engage in White Supremacy, as it assesses the South Asian tradition in terms of the tradition of White people.

Scholarship Is about Being a Student

Typical students of Yoga attempting to learn from the literature will only be treated to *W*estern *saṃskāra*-s. I bring all of this up to flag the immense hurdles that students face in the study of the philosophy of Yoga. If it were not already bad enough that Yogaland is an uncontrolled exercise of *W*AC where the South Asian tradition is appropriated to ritualize *W*estern political organization derived from Plato and Aristotle (see Chapter 2), the academic study of South Asia is, with very few exceptions, even worse. For here we find the authority of the academy directed to reifying the *W*est as the explanatory platform for South Asia. It is for this reason that, when students ask, I can almost never recommend anything worth reading or pursuing in this field. To really do justice to the wisdom of the *Yoga Sūtra*, we need to reject interpreting it and focus on explicating it. This in itself is a radical decolonial act, which rejects the methodology of colonialism: interpretation. This further reveals that activism and moral philosophy – what is often called social justice – are simply part of the content of the *Yoga Sūtra*. Yoga is a process of ethical engagement (YS I.2–4), and it ends in a moral revolution, which constitutes autonomy (YS IV.29–34).

I came to the *Yoga Sūtra* as a student of philosophy, and long before I started studying Yoga, I studied Philosophy. This study began when I was 19 and an undergraduate student of Philosophy. I learned the following then. Bad students of Philosophy will do anything to avoid unpacking and explicating the arguments of what they read. This is because they try to interpret it, which in and of itself disables reasoning. Against the backdrop of the frustration of not being able to follow the argument, they will try to interpret it in light of cultural expectations, or they will look to a *secondary* work, which talks about the primary text and is designed to be more accessible. They will read commentaries instead of original texts. This is frowned upon in Philosophy. It is one thing to read a scholarly secondary account of Plato or Kant. No serious philosopher will regard the secondary commentary as a replacement for diving into the original text. Yet bad students of Philosophy do this: they are unable to read the original text *because* they try to interpret it. The methodology of the bad Philosophy student is par for the course in Western Yoga Studies.

Bad Students of Philosophy: Welcome to Yoga Studies

If we were to explicate the *Yoga Sūtra*, we would observe that it articulates a basic ethical theory, which we reviewed in the previous chapter. We would also observe that the earliest commentary on the *Yoga Sūtra*, by someone known as Vyāsa, is heavily inspired by Sāṅkhya. Recall, as examined in Chapter 3, Yoga is a philosophy of choice and responsibility. Sāṅkhya denies that people are agents capable of being effective in their life. Vyāsa's commentary articulates a philosophy that contradicts Yoga. Why did South Asian philosophers write commentaries that are at variance with the original text? Historically, it was thought to be rude to claim to have an original idea, so many South Asian authors wrote commentaries on *sūtra* texts as a way to get their point across. Nowadays, many South Asian authors and translators of the *Yoga Sūtra* also have colonial trauma to contend with, which leads them to mistakenly present the *Yoga Sūtra* in ways that are palatable to Western *saṃskāra*-s. But Vyāsa wrote his commentary centuries ago and so Western colonialism is not an obvious ingredient. South Asians were not immune to *saṃskāra*-s and ego, and this apparently was how Vyāsa approached the *Yoga Sūtra* – in terms of his beliefs and worldview. He did so, however, deliberately and transparently as a commentary.

Western Indologists/Yoga Studies authors, operating with the Western *saṃskāra* or LAT, attempt to understand the *Yoga Sūtra* via Linguistics, but as

LAT leads to interpretation that disables reasoning, they are unable to understand the arguments of the *Yoga Sūtra*. And so they typically look to Vyāsa's commentary as a substitute, as it is more accessible. In expressing Sāṅkhya, it echoes the sense of passivism and lack of agency, which is an experience that interpreters have, as interpretation involves giving up on one's own autonomy via the conflation of oneself with one's beliefs. Vyāsa will hence appeal to interpreters. To emphasize, they do exactly what bad Philosophy students do: they avoid explicating the primary text and rely instead on secondary material or cultural interpretive resources.

Edwin Bryant,[5] for instance, *begins* his study of numerous commentaries and the *Yoga Sūtra* with the claim that the *Yoga Sūtra* was codified by Vyāsa and we have to read it thus (pp.xxxix–xl). Bryant is unusual in citing me and my approach as correct at the end of his investigation (pp.465–466) – but that contradicts where he begins. David Gordon White[6] claims that being a critical scholar of the *Yoga Sūtra* is just about reading commentaries, in stark contrast to what being a critical scholar amounts to in Philosophy. Philipp Maas,[7] a very influential Western Indologist, claims: (a) it's not his fault he can't understand the *Yoga Sūtra*, the *sūtra*s are too short (it's the text's fault, not his), and (b) in order for the text to be 'interpreted convincingly', we require cultural cues and information to understand the *Yoga Sūtra*, which leads him to the conclusion that Vyāsa's commentary was actually written by Patañjali to elucidate his *Yoga Sūtra*. Maas is unusual for trying to turn his incompetence in understanding into evidence of his innocence: as though his not being able to understand the *Yoga Sūtra* is not evidence of his inability to read Philosophy but a fault of the text. Moreover, Maas is ignorant of the fact that attempting to understand a philosopher according to cultural expectations is a way to kill the philosopher. That's exactly what happened to Socrates (as we examined in Chapter 2). So trying to understand the *Yoga Sūtra* by way of cultural explanations is to make it drink hemlock. Maas's most egregious error is the expectation that the *Yoga Sūtra* has to be 'interpreted convincingly'. Interpretation, the methodology of narcissism and colonialism, is incompatible with understanding Philosophy, as the latter requires explication – reasoning and thinking. As we saw in Chapter 3, interpretation focuses on the truth of isolated claims, while logic is concerned with inferential support. Maas's inability to understand the *Yoga Sūtra* is hence a straightforward outcome of the inappropriate (albeit ancestral) methodology he chooses: interpretation.

In opting to read the *Yoga Sūtra* in light of a commentary, he is opting for the shortcut of the bad Philosophy student.

Here is an analogy. Imagine if I, as someone with no training or competence in physics, were to announce that formulas of some famous work in physics are simply too short to understand and so one requires some cultural evidence as to their significance. I thereby construct an elaborate argument that a blog post online is authored by the author of the formulas and so we should use the blog to understand the formulas. Who would take me seriously? No one – because I lack the White privilege that would render my incompetence into the norm. In saying that the formulas are not intelligible because they are too short, I am admitting – confessing – my professional incompetence as a physicist. But it is certainly remarkable that this has been normalized in the study of Indian philosophy. Authors in Western Indology routinely confess their inability to understand South Asian uses of 'dharma' and to understand professional academic South Asian philosophy, like the *Yoga Sūtra,* as though that's the fault of the South Asian source.

Aside from the comedy of errors that we find in Yoga Studies where people without embarrassment call Vyāsa's commentary an 'auto-commentary' on the *Yoga Sūtra*, there are two problems with this. First, it's based entirely on an incapacity to actually understand the *Yoga Sūtra*. So there's no way for these folks who can't read the *Yoga Sūtra* to know whether Vyāsa's commentary agrees with the *Yoga Sūtra*. Second, even if the commentary was written by the same author of the *Yoga Sūtra*, it doesn't follow that it says the same thing. Philosophers are people: they can change their mind or be inconsistent.

BOOK 1: *SAMĀDHI-PĀDA*

What I have learned over the years is that people who adopt Western *saṃskāra*-s can fake an understanding of Western philosophy because that's where they get their *saṃskāra*-s from – to an extent. It doesn't allow any deep understanding of the implications of the Western tradition, but it does allow sounding like one understands what is transpiring in a Western philosophical text. But this is a microcosm of the politics of Western colonialism. Western colonialism treats the West as the only thing there is to know, and then people who operate with inherited *saṃskāra*-s from this tradition can (kind of) fake their way through life because they say the kinds of things said in this tradition. This makes them seem credible. So even when they admit their incompetence (say as in the case of Maas), as long as this admission is based on something central to the *W*estern tradition (like the need to interpret convincingly), they will be treated as authorities by others who share this White privilege or wish to share it by renouncing their BIPOC identity. This is a phenomenon observable throughout Yogaland, where undertrained, incompetent nonexperts teach Yoga – and what they teach is whatever they believe. To actually teach and learn Yoga, the philosophy, we have to appreciate how it is an explicit contribution to a host of philosophical debates of which moral philosophy is front and centre. That requires going beyond Yoga to learn about many options. My goal in this book is to share this knowledge while sparing the student the work of doing this research from scratch. But in sharing this knowledge I am also making clear the work the reader needs to do to understand Yoga. This is unusual. What is more normal in a *W*esternized world is the prioritization of White privilege. Students who share the White privilege of their selected teacher feel a bond with their 'teachers', for they exude the same normalized incompetence as them. Ignorance loves company. In this realm, teachers are selected because they are relatable as possessors of the same or similar *saṃskāra*-s. What is erased by this White privilege is the BIPOC philosopher. In this case, the normalized incompetence of the *W*estern tradition is treated as the starting point for serious discussion on what BIPOC philosophers have to say. And then, instead of explicating Patañjali, we try to interpret him convincingly.

It is easy to get distracted by the focus on the *W*est and the White privilege it creates and miss the insight Yoga provides. The mechanism of this normalized incompetence is the life based on *saṃskāra*-s. People from colonized traditions can and do have their own version of this problem. It is however a blessing for South Asians that if they were to actually rely upon ancestral *saṃskāra*-s it might lead them to consider explicatory criticisms of the *saṃskāra*-based life as the ancient philosophies of South Asia frequently criticized this practice. Though, in reality, this is not easy, for it requires giving up on the *saṃskāra*-s that inform us about anti-interpretive practices. Egotism that relies upon interpretive practices creates fear that prevents people from revolutionizing their lives. It manages this as it convinces the self that the place of interpretation is safe (YS 2.3, 2.9).

I didn't have these *W*estern beliefs as part of my outlook growing up though my Philosophy education was mostly *W*estern. So when I came to study Philosophy, I had to learn how to explicate in a hurry. But this was actually an advantage. It would seem like White privilege is an advantage but as an interpretive practice it prevents one from learning how to reason. I learned that with logical skills I could approach *any* philosophical text and eventually understand it *on my own*. This choice to use logic instead of belief led me to explicate a challenge: how can we translate texts like the *Yoga Sūtra* at all?

What I learned in my PhD research in preparation for my dissertation was that translation is a specialized activity that requires knowledge that goes beyond merely knowing the source (original) language and the target (translated) language. Translators specialize in *kinds* of texts, or genres. That is because what is translated are texts of a certain genre, like Philosophy, or Chemistry, and each such text is composed of *translation units* – the smallest unit to be translated as a whole. It could be a sentence, a paragraph, or a *sūtra*. A good translator hence *reconstructs* the original text with new linguistic resources. And so long as the corresponding translation units are equivalent relative to genre-specific considerations, the translation is successful. I called this *text type semantics*. This analysis of translation shows that the ordinary LAT-based account leads to problems as it confuses the meaning that transcends languages with linguistic meaning, when the meaning that transcends languages and cultures in translation has to do with disciplinary practices that define genres. As I was formulating my defence of this position, I took it upon myself to translate the *Yoga Sūtra*. What I had already formulated given my knowledge of Philosophy is that it (Philosophy) is a specific kind of text that uses words like 'morality', or 'dharma', 'knowledge', or '*pramāṇa*', reality, or '*tattva*' to articulate controversial theories. I call these *key philosophical terms*: they are terms used by every philosopher in weird ways that reflect their own theories. So a successful translation of a philosophical text preserves the structure that allows for its explication of these key terms. But it was from Patañjali that I started to learn an essential point: whatever your approach to understanding, it has to allow for a principled and disciplined approach to the data that should allow different people with different perspectives to converge on the same conclusions about the data. In being disciplined, we make space for ourselves as individuals. If we are undisciplined, we collapse the distinction between what we are perceiving and ourselves and then make everything about our ego. This is in effect what the opening lines of the *Yoga Sūtra* (YS I.2–4) teach us. And in time, I was able to credit Patañjali with the principled approach to translation I defend.

Thinking about translation units made me appreciate a *sūtra*. A *sūtra* text is composed of aphorisms, also called *sūtras*, which use polysemous words on purpose. It uses words with many meanings to condense many ideas into a short sentence. The word 'vṛtti' for instance that is central to the definition of Yoga (YS I.2), and also plays a role in the inventory of topics that Yogis have to be aware of, has several meanings. The usual approach is to pick and choose meanings according to the interpretive outlook of the 'translator'. Usually, 'vṛtti' is translated as 'wave', or 'disturbance', or 'influence'. But it also means *ethical behaviour* and to my (non)surprise, the moral philosophical importance of this word is usually left out of translations, for no good explicatory reason. What I endeavoured to do in my translation was hence to treat each *sūtra* as a translation unit and to produce a corresponding English unit that captured the various meanings, organized for their explicatory or philosophical significance.

Yoga as Metaethics and Meta-Explanatory Choice

The first *sūtra* of the text is much like the opening line of any *sūtra* text: it's a formal introduction. Here, Yoga is described as something that we have to dive into. I translated the further lines (YS I.2–3) thus:

> Yoga is the control of the (moral) character of thought.
> Then, the seer can abide in its essence.

Yoga is about taking responsibility for ordering and relating to what we experience so it *respects* our autonomy and independence, which is an ethical concern. This allows us to know. Failing that, we simply allow what we experience to influence us (YS I.2–4). Explication is a version of Yoga, for when we engage in explication, we elucidate a controversy and create room for us to evaluate it. Otherwise, we relate to what we can contemplate via propositional attitudes, whether belief, hope, or fear. In other words, when we fail to engage in Yoga, we interpret. And this leads us to be influenced by our propositional attitudes instead of organizing our thoughts and experiences.

What follows in the *Yoga Sūtra* is a discussion of what we need to appreciate as part of the practice of Yoga. Specifically, we need to make clear the various *vṛtti*-s that we must come to terms with. The *vṛtti*-s are influences that will influence us if we do not influence them. This includes: the epistemic or what is related to knowledge (*pramāṇa*), illusion, verbal delusion, sleep, and memory (YS I.5–6). What is related to knowledge is threefold: perception, inference, and the literature (*āgamāḥ*). When we practise Yoga, we do not let these influence us. We rather control or influence these factors to protect our autonomy. And hence, when we've completed the transformation necessary for a successful practice of yoga, we are in a state of autonomy (*kaivalya*). And the transition from failing to practise to successfully practising is an ethical transformation that involves getting rid of selfishness in all contexts (YS IV.29).

Let us take a couple of examples to flush this basic idea of Yoga out. Yoga as defined in the opening lines of Book 1 is really a *methodology* of data processing. It is also an account of what the options are for moral inquiry, which is the part of Philosophy called 'metaethics'. Explication, as noted, is what we do when we practise Yoga, for in responsibly processing the data, we render ideas, thoughts, and arguments *explicit* and hence something we are able to understand. The failure to practise this is interpretation, and it leads to being *influenced* by what we attend to. Western Indology and Yoga Studies are obvious examples of *failing* to engage in the explicatory practices of Yoga. And the result of this is that Western Indology and Yoga Studies are constituted by people who are *influenced* by the ancestral *saṃskāra*-s that come to them either via the inheritance of the colonizing tradition, the West, or, in some other cases, by *being* colonized by the West and then attempting to participate in this colonial tradition. What is clear is a *lack* of freedom and autonomy in Western Indology and Yoga Studies, evidenced in the expressions of frustration one frequently reads about the lack of South Asian claims about 'dharma' making any sense, or in the impenetrability of the *Yoga Sūtra*.

Another more dramatic example is the 2020 US presidential election. The American votes, as counted by poll workers, determined that Joe Biden won that election. Donald Trump claimed to have won that election. A significant subset of his supporters believed that he was the actual winner of the election and then used this belief to interpret what transpired. Call them Trumpies. The poll workers were explicators. Each properly submitted ballot was treated as a perspective that expressed a theory about who should win various races. The poll workers rendered explicit these choices and then tallied the votes. The winner of a race was simply who won the most votes in any race, and this was a simple deductive entailment of the tally. Trumpies, in contrast, interpreted every race in terms of their beliefs about who won. When the outcome was in accordance with Trumpy beliefs, they raised no objections. In jurisdictions that Biden won, ordinary voting paraphernalia and procedures were interpreted by Trumpies as evidence of corruption. Of course, we know, this culminated in the January 6 insurrection, when Trumpies stormed the US Capitol in an effort to disrupt the counting of Electoral College votes that would finalize the election.

The latter is a classic example of the distinction between Yoga and its opposite. When we practise Yoga, we can responsibly process the data to arrive at outcomes that we can then evaluate. This is what the poll workers did. When we fail to practise Yoga, we are *influenced* by our beliefs to extremes that undermine autonomy. The Trumpy in choosing interpretation, or anti-Yoga, had decided on a methodology that rendered them easily manipulated by a demagogue (Trump). But here, in reading the *Yoga Sūtra*, we see how: they were not in charge of the *vṛtti*-s so the *vṛtti*-s influenced them. What they saw, the arguments they considered, and the literature they read were like a Trojan Horse that undermined their independence. And so they became a function of the data they chose to take in – data like 'I won the election' said by Trump.

The similarity between the *W*estern Yoga Studies/Indology and the Trumpy seems vast. The former does not as a group mount insurrections. But *W*estern Yoga Studies/Indology functions to suppress South Asian philosophy by normalizing its interpretive approach to the data. And in this respect, the difference has less to do with *W*estern Yoga Studies/Indology not staging an insurrection but rather having already succeeded in that insurrection, which overthrew philosophical research into South Asia and replaced it with *W*estern interpretation. Or, perhaps more properly, we should say that if we do not object and stand for a principled approach to the data, the insurrection will succeed. The Yoga approach to these political forces is to observe that interpreters have already lost their autonomy. They are rather a function of the experiences of their culture that they internalize as their perspective, which they then employ in understanding. But in both cases, the attempt at understanding is a failure. They may be politically effective, but they are epistemic disasters.

The *Yoga Sūtra* proceeds to distinguish between different attempts at practice that it calls *abiding* (*abhyāsa*), which is a result of the exertion of will to maintain or create a steady state of experience (YS I.13–14). One form of this activity is commensurate with Buddhist practices, which involves detachment from desire (YS I.15–16). Another form of abiding in contrast can track individuality, which resembles a Jain approach to practice (YS I.17). Both contrast with the abiding of pure interpretation, where the only things left over are the interpretive tendencies (YS I.18). This occurs when the body itself collapses into natural influence (YS I.19). The Yogic option, however, is an abiding that follows from cultivating trust and confidence in the practice (*śraddhā*), remembrance, understanding of findings, and an understanding and insight (*prajñā*) into the self (YS I.20).

All forms of abiding are volitional – even the interpretive life. However, to endorse the interpretive life is to allow oneself to be a function of external influence. And so in defences of interpretation, we see both: on the one hand, there is a conscious choice to endorse interpretation, and on the other hand, there is a lack of rational autonomy that is a function of being influenced by external pressures. Yoga, in contrast, is the process that is driven by the individual and is successful in proportion to what they put into it (YS I.21–22).

Īśvara: The Practical Ideal

Another way to achieve the same practice of energy, engagement, and optimism is to engage in devotion to Īśvara. Īśvara is a special kind of person defined by two groups of traits: (a) it is unconstrained by its past, and (b) it is also unafflicted and not impeded by its future (YS I.23). Later in Book 2, Patañjali will represent these two sets of traits as separate practices of: (a) *tapas* (unconservatism), and (b) *svādhyāya* (self-governance). Īśvara is the practical ideal of what it is to be a person. A person is hence not defined by natural (*prakṛti*) traits, like species, sex, gender, orientation, or religious views. A person is the kind of thing that thrives given their own unconservatism and self-governance. Īśvara as the practical ideal of what it is to be a person hence accomplishes two things: (1) it allows us to value our own individuality as it is the ideal of what it is to be an individual, and (2) it allows us to connect to others who share an interest in their own individuality. So in being devoted to it, we explore Sovereignty in the abstract (which we share with others) and in our own particular case. But Īśvara also connects back to our starting approach to Yoga, where Yoga is the methodology of organizing one's relationship to what can be known so as to allow one's own independence. This contrasts sharply with the Trumpy or Western Indologist who is literally influenced by their beliefs. The interpreter lacks autonomy owing to a lack of Devotion to Sovereignty.

All learning originates with Īśvara, and hence it is the first teacher and abstraction that isn't bound by time. All learning is originally from Īśvara, for to learn is to become sovereign and independent of one's prejudices and false perspectives (YS I.25–26).

Its sound is 'Om' (YS I.27). Why? When we say 'Om' we produce a sound that saturates our senses and we thus have an experience of our own Sovereign efficacy as responsible agents. That is to experience our own Īśvara.

Having an understanding of Īśvara, Patañjali tells us, allows us to appreciate that our difficulties are *unnecessary*. There is nothing necessary about a problem. What follows is a review of many practices that can help us engage our own unconservatism and self-governance. We can, for instance, adopt what is called the *brahmavihāra* in Buddhism: this consists in adopting an appropriate response to things in life. This includes being pleased with what is correct, being compassionate to those who suffer, taking joy in what is good, and being indifferent to what is bad (YS I.33). The central practice of freeing ourselves of problems is the explicatory practice set out at the start of Book 1 and redescribed by the end of the chapter (YS I.43–46). Central to this explicatory practice is a skilled and clear intellect that respects the requirements of the self to be unconservative and self-governing. This exploratory practice in turn supports a world of diversity (YS I.47–48). Here, the *Yoga Sūtra* uses the ancient Vedic term '*Ṛta*' – the term for the cosmic moral order – to label the beneficence that follows from the practice of Yoga. When we practise Yoga, all things are corrected and rendered explicit. And this righting and rendering explicit supports people to make responsible choices.

We have already seen this. In Chapter 3, by employing explication, we were able to explicate for basic options of ethical theory. Yoga unlike the alternatives is the philosophy we need to understand all options of Philosophy. For to understand all the options of Philosophy is to explicate, which is Yoga at its most general level. By making options clear, we can understand and choose freely.

BOOK 2: *SĀDHANA-PĀDA*

Ideal Normative Ethical Practice

In Book 1 of the *Yoga Sūtra*, Patañjali introduces the ideal of Īśvara, and devotion to Īśvara, as equivalent to the practice of Yoga (YS I.20–24). The ideal of Īśvara is important, as it is not only the anchor of Yoga, the practice, but also the ideal of what it is to be a person. Persons, according to Yoga, are things characterized by *cetana* (YS I.29), which in Sanskrit not only denotes consciousness and knowledge but also the will. Persons are ultimately the masters of what they are aware of (YS IV.18). Even the trouble that people experience is a function of their own will (YS IV.9–10). Yet this state of difficulty is the opportunity to take hold of self-mastery (YS II.23). Patañjali's various comments about people hence are inextricably tied to the ideal of Īśvara. Īśvara is the ideal of what it is to be a person. Īśvara has a healthy relationship to its past, not being trapped or afflicted by past actions and choices. Īśvara is hence unconservative. And it has a healthy relationship to its future, not being limited by outcomes or psychological baggage. Īśvara hence self-governs (YS I.24). So to understand a person is not to understand it in terms of having the *abilities* of Īśvara. It is rather to appreciate its interest in the traits of Īśvara. So persons are the kinds of things that thrive given their own unconservatism and self-governance. Persons, according to this account, come in all sorts of shapes and forms: nonhuman animals and the Earth, as well as humans, are persons. We know this because if we bind or restrict these things by forcing them to be conservative in behaviour and we do not allow them to self-regulate, preventing their own self-governance, they become ill. The Yoga account of persons is hence radical. It explains in what case discrimination (telling apart, not treating or considering equally) is unjust. It is unjust when we equate a person with their natural attributes (like their species, sex, sexual orientation, gender identity, race, ethnicity, colonial identity) and not in terms of their interest in Īśvara. So if we were to identify people with, say, White, heterosexual, cis-gendered men, we could then use this interpretive standard to discriminate against all other things: the further they are from the paradigm case of cis-gendered, heterosexual, White men, the less they would be treated as persons. That's true in large measure in many places on Earth now and, to some extent, globally. But this would be wrong, on a Yoga account: it requires interpretation but it also confuses what it is to be a person with very superficial features of some persons, like their male sex, and lack of melanin, and heterosexuality. Devotion to Īśvara is hence a radical act of commitment to one's own individuality but also the individuality of people. To understand oneself in terms of Īśvara is to understand what people have in common: an interest in their own Sovereignty. So, for instance, when we criticize Western colonialism, we do so on a Yoga account because it confuses what it is to be a person with peculiar contingencies of the Western tradition. By the same token, in being devoted to Īśvara, we appreciate how people with these cultural, historical, or biological contingencies, like White men, are persons and deserve to be treated as such – which includes treating them as responsible for their choices.

Having identified a person as something with an interest in Īśvara, at the start of Book 2, Yoga is defined as a *kriyā* or activity that involves three practices. Yoga consists in the activity of unconservatism – *tapas* – one of the essential traits of Īśvara. It also consists in self-governance – *svādhyāya* – the other essential trait of Īśvara. And practising these two constitute what it is to be devoted to Īśvara. In other words, the practice of Yoga is to take the responsibility on to oneself to be Sovereign. There is no one else to lead us or to instruct us. All learning and understanding is from the ground up: a function of our own work.

Trauma

In Book 1, Yoga is defined as the broad methodology of being responsible for sorting the data so that one can appreciate the options. In Book 2, we appreciate what this activity looks like. It is an activity of being unconservative with respect to past activities, while also leaving room for choice via self-governance. When we explicate the options, we do both.

Choice has *two levels* on a Yoga account. The first level is the choice of methodology as we find laid out in Book 1. We can choose either the responsible ordering of the data or the identification with the data. The second level of choice is only available to those who choose the Yogic option. For to choose anti-Yoga, the identification with the data – interpretation – undermines our capacity to be free of our experiences and to live according to our own values. In other words, it undermines unconservatism and self-governance. The result is one of self-subjugation to a past one tries to maintain past its expiration. It's a haunting. Choosing the Yogic methodology for data sorting hence permits a second variety of choice: the choice to be free of one's past and to live according to one's values. So only the Yogi can access these two levels of choice.

Very often, people choose the option of ignorance – of interpretation. This leads to the ignorance of attempting to understand by way of our perspective: egotism. When we function with egotism, we function with an understanding of self based on our experiences. This consists in a state of being stuck and of being afflicted. If we are looking for a Sanskrit Yoga term that is equivalent to our word 'trauma' it is '*kleśa*'. It is now popular to speak about 'trauma-informed yoga'. However, it is Yoga that informs us of the origins of trauma. The idea that Yoga has to be informed by knowledge about trauma confuses Yoga with ableism, which assumes certain basic abilities that are not available to traumatized people. Then it seems like yoga instruction has to be informed by the challenges of people experiencing trauma. This way of talking about Yoga is a symptom of Western colonialism that erases Yoga as a basic moral philosophy that elucidates both right action and the results of wrong action: trauma. Hence we rather should talk instead about Yoga-informed trauma. It is our Yoga that should inform our trauma.[8] Yoga teaches us that trauma haunts us because we do not let go of an experience because we choose it as a means of self-understanding. This then leads us to use our own will to normalize this understanding (YS I.3). As a result of this ego-based life, which defines the self in terms of certain experiences, the person incorrectly believes that they are safe only in that experience, and they hence have an experience of fear at the prospect of change. This is why it is a state of being stuck (*abhi-niveśa*) (YS II.9). Hence the Yoga solution is to get us to do something radically different from being devoted to our experiences: Devotion to Sovereignty while practising its traits of unconservatism and self-governance.

Trauma on this yoga account is not the same as a bad experience. When we practise Yoga, we can have bad experiences. But in this case, we do not interpret and thereby use the experience to explain ourselves. We can hence move on from the challenge as practitioners. So there is nothing essentially traumatic about a bad experience according to Yoga. Our dog bite example from Chapter 2 is a case in point. Being bitten by a dog is a bad experience: it hurts. But it is only traumatic if we incorporate that event into our self-understanding. Critical thinking, Yoga, helps us see what is wrong with trying to formulate self-understanding on the basis of bad experiences. Our sample size of data (one's experience of dogs) is too small to come to any cogent induction about dogs. Conclusions, then, about ourselves as inextricably tied to these bad experiences are irrational and unjustified. If we widen the scope and start thinking about the experiences of persons as such, we will be able to come to interesting observations about systemic justice and privilege, but that involves deprioritizing one's own experiences. Correlatively, there's nothing intrinsically untraumatic about good experiences. People with immense social privilege who enjoy the best experiences their society can afford can and do generate *kleśa*. For instance, a White person who identifies with their place within the hierarchy of White Supremacy at the top of the heap internalizes the external politics of White Supremacy. They are happy when life affirms their White privilege. Yet they are unnerved when confronted with the reality of diversity, which does not fit their narrative. Here, our White Supremacist is haunted by the *kleśa* that comes from identifying with the external political order. They are traumatized because their own agency is directed toward attempting to normalize a conservative identity by way of a lack of self-governance. The unhinged behaviour of the Trumpy is a case in point. The vast majority of Trumpy January 6 insurrectionists were White Americans, who, given their country's history, have no experience of institutionalized racial oppression to speak of. Rather, as they identified with their privilege in the racial hierarchy of their country, they were aggrieved by the observation that this priority was not affirmed by the world or their fellow citizens.

Yoga: Nonideal Political Theory

The reality is that even if we ourselves are practising Yoga, many others are not. We have to contend with interpreters, whether the Trumpy, or the *W*estern Yoga Studies debutant, or the *W*estern Indologist. Put another way, while Yoga as a metaethical principle is set out in Book 1 (a principle that helps us understand the options of ethics) and Yoga as an *ideal* ethical theory is set out at the start of Book 2, where it is listed as three activities (*Īśvara praṇidhāna, tapas*, and *svādhyāya*), Patañjali sets out a *nonideal* political action plan, Eight Limbs of Yoga – a plan we can put into place in nonideal contexts. The *limbs* are *implementations* of Yoga. They are the response to an imperfect world that fails to operate according to Yoga. These limbs work to fortify Yogic practice as they help us recover what is lost: our space to be effective individuals. And so, as with all Yoga, there is no extra outcome that we are striving for. Yoga is the recovery of oneself. Hence, when succeed, we just have ourselves: *kaivalya*.

Hence, the first limb, called *Yama* (YS II.30–36), is a universal obligation to disrupt systemic harm (*ahiṃsā*), that reveals the fact (*satya*) of people not deprived of their requirements (*asteya*), their personal boundaries respected (*brahmacarya*), and no one hoarding (*aparigrahā*). This activism has the effect of getting opponents to renounce their hostility (YS II.36). The disruption of systemic harm is, on the Yoga account, our own divestment from the political order of oppression. When we decide not to internalize the *saṃskāra*-s of colonial traditions, we disrupt this systemic harm by disrupting our role in this order.

It is noted in Chapter 1 that M. K. Gandhi, who was responsible for formulating a mass, nationwide movement of civil disobedience that was aimed at getting the British to let go of their colonial hold on India, drew heavily from the *Yoga Sūtra* as the grounds of his political philosophy. Further, as noted, M. L. King took inspiration from Gandhi's project, and now that approach to disrupting systemic harm, founded on the *Yoga Sūtra*, is a blueprint for progressive political activism (whether Black Lives Matter, or Direct Action Everywhere). The reason that Yoga can operate as this blueprint for progressive political activism is not only its appreciation that we need a nonideal political action plan to create space for people, but also the Yoga account of what it is to be a person – something with an interest in Īśvara, that is, its own unconservatism and self-governance – cuts through natural boundaries and allows us to appreciate what we have in common with a diverse array of beings. And *all* of this goes back to the *Yoga Sūtra*. It isn't from Plato, Aristotle, or a Western philosopher that we learn about the importance of engaged politics to disrupt oppressive regularities. Indeed, Plato and Aristotle, and those who followed, were too busy trying to figure out how we could be convinced to obey the law. And as community was the foundation of Western political organization, Western political thinkers did not conceive of community as the foundation of oppression: they (beginning with Plato) rather tried to justify inequality as necessary for political order. This continues into the thought of Liberals, like Hobbes (who defends dictatorship) and Mill who defends racial inequality (*On Liberty* ch. 1). Indeed, one of the signs of Westernization is treating community as the basic explanation of justice. In Yoga, communities might be just, or they could be unjust. There's nothing sacred about community and we must practise so as to disrupt institutionalized oppression.

It is here in the discussion of the *Yama*-s that Patañjali sets out the activism of Yoga. This involves an insight into the trauma-based origins of systemic violence and the adherence to a different kind of practice based on the disruption of harm. So, for instance, if we were not to follow this Yogic advice, we would criticize Western Indology and Yoga Studies or the Trumpy on the basis of our beliefs. We would provide a contrary interpretation to the Yoga tradition as the grounds for complaining. But this would not actually provide an alternative to trauma-based activity. In pointing out the methodological alternative of Yoga, we are demonstrating a practice that all can participate in that does not depend upon ethnic identity or any particular set of experiences. The key to Yoga activity is that it restores us to a state of autonomous action.

So in engaging in the activism of Yoga, we are already acting in ways that are independent of external coercion.

One reason none of this is clearly appreciated is that the idea of *ahiṃsā*, or not-harm, is ambiguous and requires philosophical elucidation. A teleological position like Jainism that we looked at in the last chapter understands *ahiṃsā* in terms of its ends. So to engage in *ahiṃsā* is to not break things on this account. Buddhists too can make use of the idea of *ahiṃsā*. But for them, it will have to do with suffering, and they will consider *ahiṃsā* as something that avoids psychological discomfort. In Yoga, *ahiṃsā* is radically procedural: it is about acting in ways that depart from systemic harm. And contrary to the teleologist, the Yogi knows that this will break bad conventions and it will also amplify psychological discomfort of interpreters. The Yogi also knows (as we shall see in Chapter 6) that sometimes *ahiṃsā* means fighting in a war if that's what it takes to disrupt systemic harm. For sure, there may be discomfort in these activities, but that is a function of a problem that has festered for too long. It can't be blamed on the intervention. So White Supremacists will *feel upset* in the face of Yogic activism. But that is the fault of the egotism of the White Supremacist, not the Yogi.

Having engaged in this activism, one can then proceed to the *Niyama* (the second limb) where the practitioner commits to the three basic ideal practices of Yoga while working on being content and pure in this commitment (YS II.32).

The third limb, *āsana*, is about occupying the space that one has created via Yogic activism and practice (YS II.46–48). It is a physical commitment to relaxing and being active in the personal space of Yoga. In contemporary yoga talk, '*āsana*' is the word for postural exercise. This exercise bears a resemblance to what is discussed in the *Yoga Sūtra* to the extent that postures are ways to practise the three basic procedural commitments of Yoga. This, and all further yogic practice, happens within the context of the original activism: *Yama*.

The fourth limb is *Prāṇāyāma*, which superficially relates to practices of breath but is also described as the process of deconstructing natural barriers between oneself and the external world (YS II.51). Yoga is not about any external or extra end. It is about recovering one's space as a practical agent. And hence in controlling one's boundaries, we are taking back our control of our own personal boundaries.

The fifth limb of *Pratyāhāra* is the withdrawal of the senses from objects but also the correlative abstraction of objects from beliefs. This puts the senses under the control of the person (YS II.54–55). Having created a political space to exist, having committed to the practice of Yoga, having physically occupied that space, and having taken control of one's boundaries, now the agent decides what they will direct their attention to. This sets up possibilities of advanced practice.

The first five limbs form the core of the social aspects of Yoga's nonideal theory. While it may seem as though many of the limbs are goal oriented, they are called 'limbs' of yoga as they are means of implementing Yoga, the ultra-procedural ethical theory, both metaethically and ethically. Each limb involves the metaethical challenge of appreciating alternatives, and each exemplifies Devotion to Sovereignty (*Īśvara praṇidhāna*) and the two component practices of unconservatism (*tapas*) and self-governance (*svādhyāya*).

CONCLUSION: STOICISM AS ANTI-YOGA

Marcus Aurelius, the Roman Emperor who presided over colonized territories, was also a Stoic philosopher. In Book 4 of his *Meditations*, he makes several astounding claims. First, he argues that the reason people have problems is because they complain. Take away the complaint, and you take away the problem. He also says that we should consider that everything that happens, happens justly. In other words, if you think there is a problem with the world, you are looking at it the wrong way. This is a philosophy of non-critical acceptance that blames the individual for problems. *W*AC-ky yoga students inheriting this as part of their *saṃskāra*-s, will notice an attraction to classical Buddhism. Classical Buddhism claims that problems arise from the psychology of individuality, which desires and wants what is not possible. Reality is simply a continuity of causes and effects it calls *dependent origination*. Problems are really the fault of the individual on this account, which tries to make itself an exception against the backdrop of dependent origination. The individual's bad attitude (desire) and a failure to have correct beliefs about the world (the Four Noble Truths) is to blame. This is one explanation for why Buddhism gets confused with Yoga in Yogaland. It echoes Stoicism, in a most colonizing *W*estern moral theory, in blaming the individual's attitude and perspective for its problems.

What we are doing in our investigation is unusual in an account of Yoga and South Asian philosophy. The ordinary approach is to assume a *W*estern perspective and thereby interpret. The result is that this colonizing tradition is normalized and not the subject of complaints. Rather, South Asian philosophy as it deviates from the basics of Western *saṃskāra*-s is criticized. For the Western Indologist Yoga Studies author, the actual world, colonized by the West, is fine. The problem is the South Asian tradition that tries to make an exception of itself. Hence, it is difficult to understand.

Yoga is not the idea that everything is fine and that problems are a result of complaints or reducible to a bad attitude or because we want things. According to Yoga, problems arise because of a lack of personal independence. Recovering this independence is a public activism that assigns blame to interpretation and provides an alternative that we can all do: Yoga. Yoga-based criticism does not condemn White Supremacists to a life of White Supremacy. In identifying the choice such folks are making and the clear readily available alternative, we are teaching what is usually hushed. There is no need for the normalized nonsense we have gotten accustomed to. The problem is that we internalized this pervasive White Supremacy as normal. And this compromises our own individuality. If we do not explicitly abandon it, we use our own agency to normalize it, and this constitutes an affliction.

CHAPTER 4 REFLECTIONS

» Given that the academic literature is filled with interpretations of Yoga, how can you discern credible sources of information?

» Why is interpretation bad no matter who does it?

» What is the relationship between Yoga as defined at the start of Book 1 and Yoga as a normative practice as defined at the start of Book 2?

» How is Yoga a philosophy of activism?

» What is the difference between the Eight Limbs of Yoga as an *upāya* or remedy and the basic practice of Yoga?

» How can instruction of small 'y' yoga be a way to practise capital 'Y' yoga?

» How can yoga spaces be spaces for activism? Is it possible to responsibly teach and practise yoga in enclosed spaces without first engaging in *Yama*?

» Have you encountered Stoicism being passed off as Yoga? How would a practice based in *Yama* confront this?

» How can the first Limbs of Yoga be practised at two levels? What are the two levels, for instance, of practising *Āsana* and *Prāṇāyāma*?

» How is Īśvara, and devotion to Īśvara, different from ordinary ideas of God, and devotion to those gods?

» According to ordinary accounts of privilege, someone has White privilege (a series of advantages available only to White people) because of the external political order of White Supremacy. According to a Yoga account of political orders, to have privilege, like White privilege, one has to adopt the *saṃskāra*-s that uphold the power structure of White privilege. How does the Yogi get rid of their privilege, and why would they do that? (Hint: *Yama*-s.)

CHAPTER 5

YOGA *SŪTRA*: SELF-CARE (BOOKS 3 AND 4)

INTRODUCTION: WHY START WITH BLAME AND COMPLAINTS?

Self-care is currently commodified in Yogaland as a kind of spa treatment. Online, people claiming to peddle Yoga will offer you advice on small 'y' yoga practice as a way to take care of yourself, along with fresh juices and other interventions, like chanting. The main sign of this exercise is the idea that we need to take some special time of the day for self-care, to calm ourselves down. Self-care is significantly compromised by systemic oppression. If we adopt the Stoic approach, self-care is about erasing agitation. Much of what passes for self-care in Yogaland is motivated by this Stoicism. If I were to adopt this approach, I would be agitated by the Yoga we are exploring here, as it provides grounds for complaints. And as noted, the *WAC*-ky adoption of Buddhism as the South Asian proxy for Stoicism also plays a role in this spa version of self-care. In so far as this is an exercise of interpretation, it is also, as noted in Chapter 3, an exercise in narcissism.

The problem is that if my agitation is caused by a systemic harm, then a narcissistic focus on my attitude and desires does not address the root cause of my problems. *In fact*, if systemic harm is about my internalization of the external oppressive political order by adopting its *saṃskāra*-s, then calming myself down is a way to normalize this internalization of oppression. For instance, if we were simply not fussed by the treatment South Asian philosophy and philosophers like Patañjali get in the literature, we would be part of the normalization of that incompetence grounded in White privilege that erases Brown philosophers like Patañjali. This problem is systemic: it's not just about Patañjali and how nonexpert Western authors erase him by interpreting Yoga. Consider two interactions I have talked about on my Instagram page in 2023.

I was scheduled to teach an online course for the Kripalu Center for Yoga and Health in 2022. I'm a scholar of moral and political philosophy, as well as the South Asian tradition, and especially Yoga. I have three graduate degrees on these topics, over 50 peer-reviewed publications that overlap on these areas of specialization, two edited volumes, and two monographs to my name (this is my third!). It is hence with considerable background that I put together a course on Yoga and Activism. When it came time for Kripalu to advertise the course, they sent out an email on April 1 for a course that was to start in May. And the email contained pictures and names of all of the presenters (except two). The acknowledged presenters were female and or White. My course was listed at the bottom of the email. My name was not included, nor my picture. Instead, I was replaced by a generic (nameless) white woman. And it turns out I had company. They did the same thing to the other South Asian male presenter (Yogrishi Vishvketu (Vishva-ji)) in the same email. Kripalu did this not because (in their words) they were trying to erase me, but because they wanted to 'appeal to all of our audience'. In other words, appealing to their whole audience at Kripalu seemingly required not having two South Asian men on their programmes.

In 2020 I was scheduled to give my first of two online workshops at Yoga Alliance. I looked up the schedule and noticed that my colleague, Dr Anya Foxen (who is White and female), was also presenting around the same time as me. I noticed that on the schedule she was listed as: Dr Anya Foxen, Assistant Professor of Religious Studies and Women's and Gender Studies at California Polytechnic State University. I was described as: Shyam Ranganathan. 'Dr' was omitted and I was described as though I didn't have an institutional affiliation (Department of Philosophy, York Centre for Asian Research, York University, Toronto), which academics like Dr Foxen do. I wrote to my contact doing the scheduling at Yoga Alliance. She apologized and said that she would correct this, but my listing was merely corrected to include 'Dr' in the title: my institutional affiliation was left out. I had to escalate to Dr Kuberry (who was in charge of Standards at Yoga Alliance) and ask if this could be corrected but also if some explicit attention could be called to the matter of how BIPOC are described and advertised in Yoga Alliance events. So I had to push back twice!

I have had many other problematic experiences with 'big yoga' which would not have occurred had people explicated the options, but would occur if they interpret on the basis of the *W*estern tradition. For instance, I remember once receiving substantive criticisms of my writing from a nonexpert editorial assistant at IAYT (the International Association of Yoga Therapists), who lacked any and all academic expertise in Philosophy and Yoga but felt that she had seen enough in the world to know that I (a BIPOC scholar, philosopher, and historian of Yoga and South Asian philosophy) couldn't be correct in my writings on Yoga – even though I was the invited keynote speaker for their upcoming conference that year. This is common and expected: folks who internalize the *W*estern tradition will find what I say wrong because it does not gel with their *W*estern *saṃskāra*-s even though I am the expert and they aren't. This is White Supremacy at work, namely *W*estern *saṃskāra*-s getting in the way of understanding. In this case, the beliefs and prejudices that one gains in a *W*esternized world (which as noted in Chapter 2 are anti-philosophical) encourage overriding the knowledge of the expert philosopher. This may seem like a slightly different way to define White Supremacy as earlier I defined it as a political order created by *W*estern colonialism. But these come to the same thing as the political order is the employment of *W*estern *saṃskāra*-s as an ordering process and final explanation. True to form, *W*estern colonialism has no place for the philosopher's knowledge. That requires explicating and giving up on interpreting via *W*estern *saṃskāra*-s. But White Supremacy does value and promote the beliefs one inherits as someone whose ancestry is *W*estern. This is White Supremacy not because people engaging in this are using the colour of skin as a criterion of explanation. It is because it relies on the tradition of White people as the backdrop of explanation: Yoga the philosophy is not part of this backdrop.

Another time, Yoga Alliance was supposed to grandfather me into their certification so that I could offer continuing education training to Yoga teachers. I had to have a conversation with a person presiding over this process, who was shocked to find out that I had taken very few *āsana* classes. In her view, this meant that I couldn't be an expert on Yoga because apparently the only way to learn about Yoga is from small 'y' (colonized) yoga classes. I told her that I learned about Yoga from the ground up: by becoming a professional philosopher, a South Asianist who knew Sanskrit, and a translation expert. I learned Yoga from Patañjali and other ancient South Asian philosophical sources, from the original Sanskrit texts. This seemed to be incomprehensible to her. Though she had my CV (at the top it says that I translated the *Yoga*

Sūtra), in exasperation, she wanted to know if I at least knew what the Eight Limbs of Yoga are. Either she didn't know where the Eight Limbs of Yoga came from, or she didn't believe my CV: either way, these would not have been the outcomes had she explicated my expertise. These are outcomes that are a result of interpreting on the basis of the *W*estern tradition, with a history of *W*AC-ky yoga (as reviewed in Chapter 2). According to *W*AC-ky yoga, you can only learn about Yoga in modern YTTs. (Indeed, that's why ancient South Asian philosophers are depicted by *W*AC-ky yoga as being irrelevant. They didn't learn about Yoga in modern certified YTTs, from Platonic gurus at the top of yoga pyramids, or from Aristotelian cultural immersion. They learned about Yoga by explicating it.)

Oppression tries to convince us that a systemic harm is really our own personal problem that we need to just calm down about (YS II.3). This is a lie. Hence, self-care is ultimately a political exercise. In every case of being met with racist treatment, I had to stand up for myself, publicly, to regain my space to be myself. In some cases, this confrontation resulted in dramatic improvements. In all cases, the organizations in question apologized, and in some cases, such as Kripalu and IAYT, substantial changes were made to avoid a repetition of the discrimination I had experienced. The transformation these organizations engaged in is *to their credit* and speaks to them being organizations we should engage with. But it wouldn't have happened without me pushing back. I have a history of activity and work that is deliberate and responsible, including my academic accomplishments. To allow this to be erased would be irresponsible. Hence, in confronting and criticizing these various organizations, I could not simply throw bombs and burn bridges. In every case I have remained engaged with these organizations, and I am working to create a different future with them, where everyone involved can say that these mistakes are in the past. Yogic activism is constructive. It allows everyone to move forward past error. Yoga also teaches us that there is no perfect organization, past, or context. Everything has to be altered for the better by our activity. Yoga hence stands in sharp contrast to other moral philosophies that require that we only associate with and work with people who live up to our standards. That kind of moral narcissism ensures that nothing changes for the better.

If I think about a commonality of the authors of my marginalization, they were typically White women, who know nothing about Yoga or philosophy, employed by yoga organizations and in charge of their communications (or just random yoga teachers online who are also ignorant) having difficulty acknowledging the *unusual* expertise of a dark man. *W*AC-ky yoga likes to install South Asian men, who are known for one thing (like a style of *āsana* or meditation) as its Platonic king. It doesn't have room for the idea that learning about Yoga requires learning about a diversity of philosophy and being a successful person independently of pyramid schemes and ashrams. I, a Brown philosopher, simply don't fit into a *W*estern world.

I have come to wonder about the correlation of my treatment with the treatment that dark men receive in White Supremacy, where the dark man has to be removed, ignored, corrected, and erased to make others feel comfortable. The news of late, as I write, has been filled with accounts of Black men at the receiving end of police violence in the US. In Canada, recently, the news has reported the disproportionate rate of Black and Indigenous deaths at the hands of police. One reason that these events have resonated with me is that in the case where I was replaced by a nameless White woman for a course I was teaching, the justification had to do with attempting to present an image that made people feel comfortable and welcome. The need to erase the dark male philosopher is not so different from the academy where *W*estern Indology and Yoga Studies displays a great difficulty learning from Brown philosophers like Patañjali. Here, Patañjali is treated not as someone providing reasons for conclusions but rather as someone to be interpreted by the beliefs of White people.

My experience is part of a larger pool of data that represents how historical Brown philosophers are treated in the *W*est, where they are typically interpreted by *W*estern authors or marginalized as religious figures. But it also brings to light the ways that *W*AC-ky approaches to self-care are insufficient. Breathing exercises and fresh juices are not going to solve the infringement on my personal space I experience as a racialized philosopher. If this can happen to me, despite my profile, imagine how normalized this kind of discrimination in Yogaland is, where BIPOC participants and teachers will be treated as marginal side notes by big yoga.

Yoga helps us understand what it is to be a person and how the problem isn't White people or White women. The problem is the White Supremacy of *W*estern interpretation. And the problem with *W*estern interpretation is interpretation. Even though it is bolstered by basic commitments in the *W*estern tradition, it is bad no matter who does it. And the gift of Yoga is it helps us appreciate the error as something *distinct* from the people engaging in the mistake. So the political activism of Yogic self-care makes it possible for everyone to change their ways. But to appreciate this is to also appreciate the real history of affliction. The real history of affliction is *choosing* interpretation, or anti-Yoga. That confuses our experiences with our sense of self, and then we attempt to normalize everything in accordance with that contingent sense of self called *asmitā* (egotism).

The *Yoga Sūtra*'s first two books help us identify both the origins of harm (interpretation) and the political requirement to disrupt it. If we do not make that political space of the first five limbs, we will not create an environment in which we can care for ourselves. *Āsana* in Yoga is not running away from politics. It is about taking up the full space one creates via one's activism. What it teaches is that caring for oneself is about reclaiming one's space in one's life to be an agent (Book 1). And this involves practising agency (*Īśvara praṇidhāna* – Devotion to Sovereignty – which involves the practice of being Sovereign, which involves unconservatism – *tapas* – and self-governance – *svādhyāya*) and ensuring that public space is safe for people to engage in these practices (Book 2). So we have to nestle our own practice (as a commitment of the *Niyama*) within a wider political activism of *Yama*-s, which makes space for people. In this chapter, we will look more closely at what the third and fourth books have to teach us. The third book of the *Yoga Sūtra*, called the *Vibhūti-pāda*, has to do with the power of yoga practice that facilitates self-care. It is a practice that we do along with our political activism. The fourth book, the *Kaivalya-pāda*, is about the transformation of the practice, which ends in autonomy (*kaivalya*). This is a state of perpetual self-care and one made possible by perpetual self-responsibility. This autonomy requires appreciating our place within a public world but also the ways in which we are different from others, especially those who interpret. Before we get to examining their content, in the next section we will investigate the question: who or what are you? Yoga has a very specific response to this question that has to do with the practice of Yoga. With a clearer answer to this, we can examine the question of what it is to care for ourselves.

WHAT ARE YOU?

What are you? That is a philosophical question. There are several answers. If we look to the Western tradition, starting with Plato, the predominant answer is that you are (in part) your mind, and the word for this is 'soul'.

Little wonder then that Western thinkers inheriting a Western idea of the self as their mind are inclined to explain everything in terms of their mind: interpretation. It is on the basis of this definition of the self that selves can be distinguished according to their inherent virtues and psychological traits. According to Plato, those lacking reason as a defining feature need to be lied to as they can't appreciate reason. Plato in the *Phaedrus* theorizes that this difference in the character of the soul accounts for the differences between the gods and the rest of us. Aristotle takes this to the next level by observing that some humans, owing to the inherent state of their mind, are naturally born slaves (*Politics* 1254b16-1). As the Western tradition develops, this account of the self as including one's mind is reinvented as the Liberal idea of the self as defined by preferences, starting with Hobbes. On a Liberal model, each one of us is unique in so far as our preferences are personal, and autonomy is about being able to act on what one wants. To be sovereign on this account is to get what one wants (also, as Hobbes explores in his *Leviathan*). This was universally rejected in the South Asian tradition – though Western commentators are quick to use the idea of the soul to talk about the self. On the Buddhist account, if you are your mind, you are better off accepting that there's no such thing as you – as your mind is just dependently originating thoughts and experiences. Hence, the position has sometimes come to be known as the *anātman* (no-self) view.

From the very earliest sources of Yoga, the reduction of the self to the mind (and hence, the reduction of the self to the soul) was rejected. In the *Kaṭha Upaniṣad*, which we shall examine in greater detail in Chapter 6, the mind is the synthesis of perception and intellectual direction. In the *Yoga Sūtra*, we learn that mind is a creature of ego or the identification with a perspective (YS IV.4). According to Yoga, you are a practical agent responsible for your life. That is what it is to be a person: *puruṣa*. This is not the same as one's body, mind, senses, or intellect. When the person is in charge of their life, these various elements express a coherent whole, which is the person. Yoga is the practice of this synthesis and joining. When we are ill, our lives are fragmented into aspects of ourselves, such as body, mind, or intellect.

In order to understand yourself, you need to respect yourself as an abstraction from the contingencies of your life, which you can then use to evaluate yourself. This is implicit in many discussions of Yoga's philosophy, such as the *Upaniṣad* and the *Bhagavad Gītā* (which we will examine in the next chapter). But we also find this in the *Yoga Sūtra*, where the self is idealized as its own master (*sva-svāmī*, YS II.22), but also ideally standing on its form (*svarūpa-pratiṣṭhā*, YS IV.34) and abiding in its form (*svarūpe'vasthānam*, YS I.3). The most explicit acknowledgement of the self as an abstraction from its life is the formulation of the accomplished state of Yoga as *kaivalya*: isolation, autonomy. This state of *practical* isolation from external influence is something we come to upon an ethical cleansing (*dharmameghasamādhi*). Sovereignty on the Yoga model isn't merely the freedom to implement what one wants. It is unconservatism and self-governance. It is a healthy and responsible relationship to one's past, where old habits, assumptions, and prejudices, do not rule one: this is the practice of *tapas*. And it is a healthy and responsible relationship to one's future, where one can act in accordance with the values one sets oneself: this is the practice of *svādhyāya*. The account of the self from Liberalism as the maximizer of personal preferences fails to be Sovereign – Īśvara – even when it gets to do as it pleases. One can do whatever one wants, and in accordance with one's desires, and fail to act on the basis of a healthy relationship to one's past (*tapas*) and future (*svādhyāya*).

Pursuing the Yogic idea of the self, you as a person, as something that should be cared for and celebrated also brings into sharp relief the very common Western interpretation of Yoga. The opening lines of the *Yoga Sūtra*, which are about ordering your mental life as a project of ethical respect for persons, are interpreted as an exercise of self calming. In a Westernized world, this assumes a Stoic backdrop, where the problem is not the politics of colonialism but your attitude toward things – accordingly, everything is fine, the problem is your agitation or anxiety. This is an interpretation – an explanation in terms of belief – of the world, and interpretation, as noted, is methodological narcissism. Yoga, in sharp contrast, does not depend upon a belief but is about what we *ought to do*. We can fail, but to engage in the activity requires vigour (*vīrya*) and optimistic commitment (*śraddhā*) (YS II.20). Unlike the Jains who see strength (*vīrya*) as an essential trait of the person and something that is confused by activity, in Yoga, it's something we do, to create a life that respects us as agents. This brings us to several important features of Yoga, the basic moral theory.

The ethical practice of Yoga is about *reclaiming* our own space in our life. This is why it happens within the context of Devotion to Sovereignty. There is no *extra* motivation or thing that we accomplish via Yoga. Your outcome of Yoga is you, just you. And this is a good thing because normally the unyogic life involves confusing oneself with experiences and events. Hence, at the end of Book 4, the outcome of Yoga is depicted as *kaivalya* – isolation. Many interpret this in very strange ways to imply that the Yogi has somehow left reality, or the world, or life. But this transition to isolation happens as a function of an ethical transformation (*dharmameghasamādhi*) (YS IV.29–34). The *Yoga Sūtra* emphasizes this by beginning with a definition of Yoga as a transformative ethical practice that allows for personal independence (YS I.2–3) and ends there too.

Given that we are agents, on the Yoga account, we need to live a life of success, as agents. This means being an effective person. An effective person is one who is powerful and protected. Needing to live such a life is not the same as being *able* to live such a life. The Yoga ideal of our lives is not descriptive of some type of ability. It rather points to what we ought to have as persons: namely our own life, which is an outcome of ourselves. How do we do this?

There are three levels of Yogic practice. First, there is the basic practice of being committed to explication, and the responsible life or organizing the data, so that one's own autonomy is preserved. This is the methodological foundation specified at the start of Book 1. Then there is the normative ethical practice, of the three *kriyā*-s: unconservatism (*tapas*), self-governance (*svādhyāya*), which both happen within the context of Devotion to Sovereignty (*Īśvara praṇidhāna*) stated at the start of Book 2. But as we do not begin our practice in ideal conditions, we need a nonideal political practice: the Eight Limbs of Yoga. The nonideal practice changes public space into something that allows for us to work on the ideal practice. It does this by starting first with *ahiṃsā*: the disruption of harm of our own internalization of the external political order. So for us to engage in the practice of self-care, what the *Yoga Sūtra* calls *saṃyamaḥ* (the practice of the last three limbs), this is something we have to do with (*saṃ*) the *Yama*-s.

In Book 2 of the *Yoga Sūtra*, Patañjali explores the normative, three-part theory of Yoga as the three essential practices of *tapas*, *svādhyāya*, and *Īśvara praṇidhāna*, and then proceeds to explore the first five of Eight Limbs of Yoga. These are described as 'outer'. They pertain to the creation of public space for independent people.

The last three limbs, explored in Book 3, are grouped together as *saṃyamaḥ*. These practices create personal power for the agent. They can be used to help protect and care for the practitioner. They can also constitute a challenge, which we need to rein in as we practise Yoga.

BOOK 3: *VIBHŪTI-PĀDA*

I find many of my students get confused between two aspects of Yoga. On the one hand, Yoga criticizes doing anything for an outcome. Doing something for the sake of an outcome is Consequentialism, which is a whole other ethical theory. However, the practice of Yoga is supposed to produce very many beneficial outcomes. So then, if we are engaging in Yoga with the expectation of good things happening, aren't we failing to practise Yoga?

Yoga rejects the idea that we ought to practise yoga for some end. We ought to be putting energy into ourselves and reclaiming our own independence. But it doesn't follow from this that Yoga doesn't produce many excellent benefits. And moreover, if we understand what Yoga is, we should expect good results. The nature of the benefit of Yoga is the reclamation of one's own power and authority to live one's own life. Properly understood, the good results *are not anything extra.* It's just you. Moreover, if you make the motivation of activity some extra good, aside from yourself, you will probably fail.

Consider some analogies. If I want to get an education so I can earn good grades, then I'll probably do badly. But if I get an education because I want to learn, I'll probably earn good grades because I'll work on learning, which is required to earn good grades. If I want to learn how to play the guitar because I want to be a rock star, I'll probably stop practising because as I start I'm no rockstar, and that possibility is far from my life. So if I set being a rock star as the motivation for learning guitar, then my beginning practice will be depicted in a light of failure, and I will hence stop practising. However, if I engage in a devotional practice to the ideal of music (the Īśvara of music), I will practise music, and in time, with enough devotion, I will start to exemplify the ideal itself, and my chances of being an acknowledged musician will correspondingly increase.

Yoga hence predicts that engaging in a practice for some extraneous end undermines the success of the practice. Rather, being devoted to the practice ensures its success, but then it is done for no extra reason. And the success of the practice is just the proficiency in the practice, which is nothing aside from a more capable, powerful you. Hence, when we make being a person our concern, being devoted to the ideal of personhood, Īśvara, sets up a practice that allows us to be successful at being a person. And the result is just you and nothing else: *kaivalya*. Moreover, if we think about unusual ends, Consequentialism demotivates pursuing them. If there is a low chance of me accomplishing something (say being a rock star or a professional philosopher who gets paid for a living to do Philosophy and teach it), I should only put in effort to that end on Consequentialist grounds that is commensurate with the chances of success. And I can tell you that when I was 19 and an undergraduate student of Philosophy looking at my future, where I am now was an extremely unlikely outcome. I could look at most people who went to graduate school for Philosophy and see that they would never have a place in the academy and would have to find other work. And when I thought about the work I wanted to do, *no one was doing it*. Still, I feel alone. No one was doing decolonial research into the history of Philosophy and the academy 30 years ago when I began. If I tried to measure the work it would take to get here, where I am, in terms of the likelihood of success, I would have had to have thrown in the towel as the evidence showed that my chances of succeeding were near zero. But even now, the question of success, and what it looks like, eludes me. I keep doing what I am doing as it is a part of my practice.

This is why in Yoga we do not do things for the outcome. We do everything as a devotional practice. And this is the essence of self-care. In being devoted to Īśvara, I do not have to put energy into what drags me down – namely difficult experiences or other people's opinions. I rather put energy into being a responsible person, which has a benefit to me and others I interact with.

All of these considerations make the topic of self-care and personal work that increases personal power tricky. Patañjali acknowledges this. On the one hand, personal work that results in powers 'can help a Yogi lead an ethical life, free from disturbances' (YS III.46). On the other hand, the outcomes of this work can sometimes be extraneous and also distracting (YS III.37–38). And the Yoga point about self-care is not reducible to coping with stress. To frame self-care in terms of the reduction of suffering or stress is to change the project from one focused on the self to one focused on pain and stress. When we focus on ourselves, to be successful people, we get rid of distractions like stress and we reduce pain. But we do so as a function of being successful as persons, not because our project was about getting rid of stress and pain.

The three final limbs of the Eight Limbs are *Dhāraṇā* (often translated as 'Concentration'), *Dhyāna* (Movement, Entailment), and *Samādhi* (Conclusion). Together called '*saṃyamaḥ*', they are described as a process that occurs sequentially. First, we identify a topic of interest with *Dhāraṇā*, then we allow ourselves to be moved by its implications. This is to engage in *Dhyāna*. Finally, we come to a conclusion in *Samādhi* – one that reveals ourselves as knowers. This is a practice that can only be engaged in conjunction with the

Yama-s (the first limb of Yoga), which involve giving upon our interpretive tendences (*saṃskāra*-s) to investigate. In Book 3 of the *Yoga Sūtra*, this three-part process is reviewed as applicable to any number of topics, and each results in an increase of personal ability and power. This is not as mysterious as it may first appear. When I teach this to my students in class, I can point to any number of technological artefacts, whether smartphones or the PC that is installed in the lecture hall. These marvels were made possible because of serial and recursive applications of *saṃyamaḥ*. People decided a topic was worth investigating, followed its implications, and arrived at conclusions that constituted an increase in capacity. For ourselves, we can apply this practice to almost any topic and come away with an increased power and ability. And the reason this works is that the power that we gain is a function of increased understanding and awareness, and this is a result of our own work.

In my own case, applying *saṃyamaḥ* to the academy and its representations of BIPOC intellectual traditions led me on a series of research journeys. The *Samādhi* at the end of this inverts the usual power structure. Usually, Western interpretation is treated as though it sets the boundaries for investigation. In my own application of *saṃyamaḥ* to this, I learned *its* limitations. That gives me power over it as I don't have to understand myself in terms of Western beliefs. All of us, with practice, can apply *saṃyamaḥ* to constraints in our lives so that we gain power over them and we do not have to internalize them.

The Three *Guṇa*-s

As far as knowledge is concerned, directing *saṃyamaḥ* to the importance of oneself allows an insight into the distinction between the quality of illumination and buoyancy (*sattva*) and yourself as a *puruṣa* that is absolutely distinct (YS III.36).

Both Yoga and Sāṅkhya analyse nature (*prakṛti*) into three *guṇa*-s. The word '*guṇa*' stands for a characteristic. The canonical words for these three qualities are: (a) '*sattva*', (b) '*rajas*', and (c) '*tamas*'. The words used in Sāṅkhya and Yoga texts for these three characteristics are not exactly the same. The distinction is between: (a) an information or data aspect of nature, (b) an active aspect of nature, and (c) a still or inert aspect. The *Sāṅkhya Kārikā* distinguishes between: (a) pleasure (*prīti*) and illumination (*prakāśa*), (b) pain (*aprīti*) and actuation (*pravṛtti*), and (c) indifference (*viṣāda*) and restraint (*niyamārtha*) (SK 12–13). In the *Yoga Sūtra*, we find a slightly different way of describing or labelling these three properties: (a) illumination (*prakāśa*), (b) activity (*kriyā*), and (c) inertia (*stithi*) (YS II.18). The difference in description is important. Sāṅkhya assumes a passive state of observation as the proper and limited role of the self (person). Activity here is something that happens to us and that can hurt. In Yoga, in contrast, we are encouraged to retake our role in our life as the primary explanation. This involves agency. Hence, the active is redescribed not as pain but *kriyā*, which is the same term used to identify Yoga as an ideal practice in Book 2.

Recently, the neurologist Stephen Porges came up with what he calls Polyvagal Theory, a theory of the functioning of the autonomic nervous system that will seem very familiar to students of Yoga.[1] Traditionally, the parasympathetic nervous system was thought to have one function: to calm. And this balanced out the sympathetic system that is active. Porges's theory claims that the parasympathetic system has two states. On the one hand, there is an aware, light, social state (*sattva*), and on the other hand, it also has a state of bringing an organism into a state of inertia (*tamas*). And this then contrasts with the sympathetic system that has the job of activity (*rajas*).

What Porges notes is that when we are well, we are able to move through these various states of the nervous system as needed. When we are ill, the *sattvic* state (what he calls 'ventral vagal') shuts down and then we are in *rajas* modes of fight (sympathetic) or flight. And in extreme cases, the sympathetic system can shut down and then we are in a state of collapse (*tamas*) (what he calls 'dorsal vagal'). This is a Yogic model of health, for it does not equate health with any particular natural state. It rather treats health as an outcome of responsible agency. But surprisingly, it also makes use of a distinction that was already known to philosophers in the Yogic tradition. It should hence not be a surprise that Patañjali acknowledges that the powers practice can be accomplished not only by the genetic endowment, chants (which engage higher functioning of the nervous system), and *tapas* (the activity of our own Yoga practice) but also herbs (YS IV.1). All of these can be utilized to help us move through various states as needed. So for the puritans who avoid caffeinated drinks like coffee and tea because they think it's unyogic: why? As long as we are dynamically in control of our functioning, a good drink or a cup of coffee can be part of the project.

Book 3 is in many ways an exploration of the powers we get by moving through various natural states. And the acknowledgement that we are distinct from these natural states (YS III.50) is an important part of reclaiming our own health and power. This means that we appreciate, in theory, that we are not exactly the same as our body, which is natural in every way (YS III.44). The point of a Yogic practice is to take charge of the natural aspects of our life, like our body, and make them personal. And this transformation is a matter of activity. Self-care is hence not reducible to any one particular activity but rather the freedom and responsibility to move through differing natural states in accordance with one's requirements as a responsible agent. The sedative approach to Yoga, seeking to calm ourselves down, is a deep confusion.

BOOK 4: *KAIVALYA-PĀDA*

Book 4, the book of Isolation or Autonomy, is a retrospective of Yogic practice. This chapter is easily misunderstood if we think Yoga is an exercise in Consequentialism. Consequentialism claims that the ends justify the means. The end of practice, *kaivalya*, isolation, will hence seem like something different from the practice, which justifies doing Yoga. Consequentialist thinking about *kaivalya* will hence imagine it as an escape from life, and many will wonder whether it is possible to attain this end given the challenges of living. But this is a deep confusion. *Kaivalya*, or isolation, is our life when our life is simply ourselves and nothing else. When we fail to live in accordance with Yogic perfection, our life is characterized by a failure to appreciate the depth of our own responsibility for our life.

When we do not own our responsibility in life, we make choices and then forget about them. Nature then returns the fruits of these choices to us – like when we leave the stove on and forget about it. Nature will boil or burn down whatever is in the pot and might start a fire. And what outcome arises as a result of our forgotten activity is a matter of natural potential. Hence, nature is like a farmer that tends to all natural events (YS IV.3).

The big obstacle to appreciating our responsibility is the mind. The mind (which is like a mirror that reflects) is a creation of the internalization of experiences, which then sets up a perspective as a way of understanding (YS IV.4). Mind here functions as representation, or theory. It is how we interpret the world. It simply reflects what we attend to (YS IV.24). But that makes it a bit like a rear-view mirror. If we look into it, what it shows us is what is behind us, or in front of the mind. If we use it to look forward, it can reflect what we see, but that reflection displaces where it actually is. When we practise Yoga, we organize the use of the mind to allow our own autonomy in the way that when we employ mirrors responsibly, say when we are driving, we are able to individuate ourselves from other objects we perceive and reflect on via our mirrors (YS IV.18). We can use our mind to see ourselves (YS IV.22) or ourselves in relationship to other things (YS IV.23). And that means that we do not rely upon a perspective to get about in life. If we can use the mind to perceive the distinction between ourselves and other things (like a mirror) then we are not impinged upon (YS IV.25). We act. Ordinarily, when we rely upon the mind, we are in the realm of memory (what is behind us, what we hold on to), and *saṃskāra* (interpretive tendencies), and there is no beginning to this as will is eternal (YS IV.9). This way of thinking of history is very different from the story-book, narrative approach that we are familiar with. According to the story-book version, there is some agent, like God, that begins everything, and before that there was nothing. That's not how South Asians thought about history, in part because they thought about the past and the future as real. The past is how we got to the present, and the future is the moral character of our choices (YS IV.12). If we can employ our mind to explicate, then we move into isolation (YS IV.26). And if we apply *saṃyamaḥ* to ethical questions, we come to a very important kind of *Samādhi*: the *dharmameghasamādhi*. This is the ethical (dharma), cleansing (*megha* – which means cloud) *Samādhi* (YS IV.29). This is the height of yogic practice. It is characterized by an abandonment of 'selfish desires in all contexts and the ever presence of discriminative knowing'. In other words, it is a state of practice free of the narcissism of interpretation. This officially initiates *kaivalya*, where the practitioner stands on the power of knowing (YS IV.34).

YOGA: THE ETHICAL PRACTICE

The *Yoga Sūtra* begins by providing a metaethical distinction between two approaches to data processing. One of these is Yoga, which has to do with making everything explicit. The other is interpretation. The latter violates logic, is ignorance, and creates ego. In Book 2, Patañjali articulates a definition of Yoga as an ideal practice, and this practice is an activity. Book 2 also initiates a distinction of how we can engage in a nonideal practice: the Eight Limbs of Yoga. The first five limbs are explored in Book 2: these have to do with converting social space into something friendly to the practice of Yoga. The last three limbs of personal care are discussed in Book 3. By the time we get to Book 4, these themes are connected, and the perfection of this practice is described as an ethical transformation: *dharmameghasamādhi.* And this transformation is the condition of our autonomy: *kaivalya.* In this case, we are the full explanations of our own life. We no longer offload choices and decisions onto nature only to have them given back to us in surprising and dangerous ways. Our anticolonial investigation of Yoga depends upon the Yogic distinction between explication and interpretation. The latter is ignorance and the cause of much difficulty. Yoga retaught as a practice of pacifying ourselves is the colonialism that we leave behind as we practise Yoga.

CHAPTER 5 REFLECTIONS

» How is personal affliction a function of systemic harm?

» In what way is the personal care of *saṃyamaḥ* (*Dhāraṇā*, *Dhyāna*, and *Samādhi*) something that we have to do along with Yama (the first limb of Yoga)?

» Describe the three components of *saṃyamaḥ* in your own words. How can we employ them to increase our personal strength?

» What is *kaivalya*? How does abandoning interpretation help us achieve this state?

» What does the difference in the way Sāṅkhya and Yoga describe the qualities of nature tell us about the Yoga approach to life?

» If the past and the future are real, how can we make sense of ourselves?

» How can doing things for oneself, like, say, having a juice or engaging in small 'y' yoga, be part of self-care on a Yoga account? How can these be an outcome of *saṃyamaḥ*?

» Why is the pacification version of yoga wrong as a way to practise Yoga?

» In Yoga, when we stand up for ourselves, we are actually making room for others too. How is self-care also good for others?

» In Yoga, when we take a stand for ourselves, how do we make future cooperation possible with people who have harmed us?

CHAPTER 6

TAKE THE FIGHT TO THE PROBLEM: *BHAGAVAD GĪTĀ* AND YOGA

INTRODUCTION

The *Bhagavad Gītā*, a discussion and lecture on moral (dharma) philosophy, is an essential source for the philosophy of Yoga. What Kṛṣṇa teaches in this dialogue under the heading of '*Bhakti Yoga*' is essentially the same as what we find as Yoga in Patañjali's *Yoga Sūtra*. Understanding this philosophy is challenging in part because of a colonial predilection to treat it as a stand-alone book. Traditionally, philosophers such as Śaṅkara and Rāmānuja have written commentaries on the *Bhagavad Gītā*. But they knew that it was merely one part of a wider epic known as the *Mahābhārata*. And as it is a dialogue between characters who have a history in the epic, treating it as its own stand-alone text is a recipe for not understanding it. Also, under British colonialism, South Asians who were told they were Hindus by the colonizer increasingly felt the need to live up to colonial expectations of religions having holy books, like the Bible or Quran. Many Hindus have identified the *Gītā* as their holy book, which can be used in official swearing-in ceremonies for instance.

In addition to needing to appreciate what has transpired in the earlier chapters of the *Mahābhārata* to understand the *Bhagavad Gītā*, one needs some further background. First, the teacher in the *Gītā*, who delivers lessons on Yoga philosophy, is Kṛṣṇa. Kṛṣṇa in turn is an incarnation (*avatāra*) of Viṣṇu. Viṣṇu and his consort Lakṣmī are canonically depicted resting on the

Cosmic Serpent, Ādi Śeṣa, and all three of them float over an ocean of external influence. As South Asians did not have the LAT, they were not restricted by the idea that Philosophy has to be explored linguistically. And so they were free to explore their philosophical ideals in art. Temple idol worship is hence part of this aesthetic exploration of philosophical ideals. These three deities are the three *kriyā*-s of Yoga – the basic three practices outlined at the start of Book 2 of the *Yoga Sūtra* – floating over an ocean of external mental influences, which is how Yoga is described (metaphorically) at the start of the *Yoga Sūtra* (YS I.2–4). This would have been obvious to people in the tradition, way back before colonialism. It is something that we have to piece together by decolonizing our understanding of South Asia.

As noted in Chapter 2, Ādi Śeṣa – the Cosmic Serpent with many perspectives – is *Īśvara praṇidhāna* (Devotion to Sovereignty). What it is to be devoted to Īśvara is to take on the practice of being sovereign, which means that there is no longer any external Īśvara that one has to obey. Rather, Īśvara disappears, and instead one has to care for the two component practices of being Sovereign: unconservatism (*tapas*) and self-governance (*svādhyāya*). Hence, Ādi Śeṣa – *Īśvara praṇidhāna* – supports the two further procedural ideals. Viṣṇu is *tapas*, or unconservatism: he is depicted with different manifestations of his activity, such as the disk, that do not constrain him. Lakṣmī is typically depicted as a lotus sitting on herself: she is hence *svādhyāya*, self-governance. As Patañjali notes in the *Yoga Sūtra*, a bond with one's chosen values is a result of *svādhyāya* (YS II.44) and so she is depicted as choosing and bonding with her chosen value: Viṣṇu. Viṣṇu, Lakṣmī, and Ādi Śeṣa form one group of procedural ideals that various traditions of Bhakti/Yoga are organized around. The other important set of values includes Śiva with his partner Śakti. He is the ideal experiencer, and she is the range of those experiences. She hence has a benign, attractive expression (Pārvatī), a fierce but attractive expression (Durgā), and a horrific and fierce expression (Kālī).

Whereas Viṣṇu is traditionally associated with *procedural* philosophies that prioritize right doing over good outcomes, Śiva, in contrast, is associated with *teleological* philosophies that prioritize good experiences over right actions. Of the four ethical theories – Virtue Ethics, Consequentialism, Deontology, and Yoga/Bhakti – the former two are teleological, whereas the latter two are procedural. Yoga/Bhakti is *the most* procedural of the four as it does not define the right thing to do in terms of the good (which Deontology does). Rather, it defines the right as devotion to the procedural ideal of the

Right: Īśvara. (For a review, see Chapter 3.) Viṣṇu turning up to deliver a lecture on Yoga's moral philosophy is hence no coincidence.

The various stories of Viṣṇu and his companions are thought experiments about the entailments of these three procedural values in differing contexts under differing pressures. The thought experiment begins with a visit to Viṣṇu by the four Kumaras, who are eternally youthful practitioners of Yoga/Bhakti. When they arrive they are met by Viṣṇu's two gatekeepers – Victory and More Victory/Jaya and Vijaya – who deny them entry to see Viṣṇu. The gatekeepers are interpreting the Kumaras on the basis of their youthful appearance, which, according to their patriarchal beliefs, renders them ineligible to visit Viṣṇu. As a result, the Kumaras curse the gatekeepers to live as demons. Viṣṇu upon learning of what has transpired appreciates that he has to be responsible for living and killing these demonic manifestations of his gatekeepers as it was he who put them in charge. There are hence numerous incarnations that follow: some of these *avatāra*-s (such as the Varāha or boar incarnation, the half-lion half-human Narasiṃha incarnation, and Rāma and Kṛṣṇa) are principally aimed at killing the demonic lives of his cursed former guards.

One of the earliest introductions to Yoga in the *Upaniṣads* also mentions Viṣṇu. This is the story of the boy Nāciketa, found in the *Kaṭha Upaniṣad*. According to the story, the boy's father had resolved to conduct a sacrifice where he gave away his possessions. The boy pesters his father with the question, 'To whom will you give me?' The father gets annoyed and says, 'To Death,' and as this is in the context of an oath to sacrifice, the boy is sacrificed to Death. When the boy arrives at Death's palace, Death is not there as he wasn't expecting the boy. Three days pass, after which Death returns. He acknowledges that he rudely stood up the boy, who should have been received properly, and hence he promises one boon for each day the boy has had to wait. Nāciketa asks: (a) to return to his father, (b) for the directions for a special sacrifice that gets one to an elevated heaven, (c) for the answer to the question of what happens to someone after they die – is that it, or is there life after death? Yama (the god of Death) grants (a) and (b) but is averse to granting (c). He tries to buy Nāciketa off with trinkets, but the boy is steadfast. Yama is super impressed and then teaches the Analogy of the Chariot.

According to Yama, the body is like a chariot in which the Self sits. The intellect (*buddhi*) is like the charioteer. The senses (*indriyāḥ*) are like horses, and the mind (*manas*) is the reins. The Enjoyer is the union of the self, senses, mind, and intellect. The objects of the senses are like the roads that the chariot travels. People of poor understanding do not take control of their horses (the senses) with their mind (the reins). Rather, they let their senses draw them to objects of desire, leading them to ruin. According to Yama, the person with understanding reins in the senses with the mind and intellect (*Kaṭha Upaniṣad* I.2). This is (explicitly called) Yoga (*Kaṭha Upaniṣad* II.6). Those who practise Yoga reach their Self in a final place of security (Viṣṇu's abode). This is the place of the Great Self (*Kaṭha Upaniṣad* I.3). There is no evil here.

This is a remarkable dialogue, as it explains that Death, the loss of control, comes in two forms. First, there is the ordinary way this occurs as an event that happens to us. This is Death as a misfortune. Then there is Death as a loss of control to oneself: this is to live life after facing Death. This is Yoga. That Death is named 'Yama' and this is also the term for the first limb of Yoga is no accident. Loss of control to oneself is essential to navigating public space where everyone's boundaries are respected. But this dialogue is also important for signalling Viṣṇu – *tapas* – as where we're heading as we practise Yoga and in bringing to light the chariot as a model. The *Bhagavad Gītā* makes use of this chariot model and installs Kṛṣṇa – Viṣṇu – as the intellect (charioteer) that will guide Arjuna. Kṛṣṇa here adopts the position of Īśvara.

With this introduction, we have set the stage for the *Bhagavad Gītā*. It is not only a continuation of a story in the *Mahābhārata*, it is also a continuation of the kinds of stories that figure Viṣṇu and his companions in articulations of the philosophy of Yoga. In the next section, we will review the plot events that led up to the *Bhagavad Gītā*. In the third section, we will consider Arjuna's lament at the start of the *Gītā*. In the fourth section, we will consider Kṛṣṇa's three responses. In the closing section, I will briefly address the issue of caste, which figures in many discussions in the *Gītā*.

THE GAME OF DICE

The *Mahābhārata* (India's largest epic) follows the fratricidal tensions and actual war of two groups of cousins: the Pāṇḍavas, five brothers including Arjuna and led by Yudhiṣṭhira, all sons of Pāṇḍu; and the Kauravas, numerous, led by Duryodhana, all sons of Dhṛtarāṣṭra. Dhṛtarāṣṭra, who is older than Pāṇḍu and first in line for the throne, is blind and hence marginalized in royal succession. Pāṇḍu is the first to have a son, Yudhiṣṭhira, so his descendants will inherit the kingdom. Pāṇḍu dies prematurely, and Dhṛtarāṣṭra becomes king as the sole suitable heir, as the next generation are still children.

Pāṇḍu's sons are decent people and good warriors, but their virtues are also their weaknesses. The Kauravas lack integrity and are less skilled in battle. Despite the Kauravas' attempts to kill them, the Pāṇḍavas compromise and defer to their relatives, easing their conflict. When the Pāṇḍavas accept an invitation to play a Kaurava-rigged dice game, they gamble their freedom, and things get worse. As warriors, the Pāṇḍavas cannot resist the challenge of the dice game, as brave warriors are not supposed to shrink from challenges. But after losing everything, they gamble away their common wife, Draupadī, in the hope of recovering their losses. She correctly excoriates all in attendance and the Pāṇḍavas for gambling her – even after they lost their own freedom. As a result, she is publicly sexually abused by the Kauravas in the hall where the game occurred. *No one* present intervenes. Yet Dhṛtarāṣṭra, the Kauravas' dad, who witnessed the whole event, including Draupadī being gambled away, does nothing – that is, until Draupadī cries over being harassed. He then nullifies the game. But they play another round. The Pāṇḍavas lose and must spend 14 years in exile, and be incognito for the final year, and if they are exposed, spend 14 more years in exile. After completing this, the Pāṇḍavas return to recover their half of the kingdom, but the Kauravas refuse to give them any space so they can support themselves. The Pāṇḍavas make every effort to reconcile but the Kauravas are intransigent. War is the only option left. Alliances, loyalties, and professional duties are publicly accounted for, and the two sides agree to fight on a battlefield.

Kṛṣṇa is a common cousin to both sides. As allegiances are finalized, both parties approach Kṛṣṇa for help. Kṛṣṇa offers himself or his army. The Kauravas choose his army. The Pāṇḍavas choose Kṛṣṇa. Kṛṣṇa agrees to be the charioteer of Arjuna, who is an excellent archer.

In the *Mahābhārata*, the Pāṇḍavas follow conventional moral standards for people of their station and occupation, including taking on risky public challenges. *Conventional morality* is the morality of good character traits (like the courage of warriors to play dice – a Virtue Ethical concern), engaging in activities with a promise of a good outcome (like winning at dice – a Consequentialist concern), and agreeing to be bound by good rules of procedure (like the rules that constitute the Game of Dice – a Deontological concern). The Pāṇḍavas' imprudence is a result of their Virtue Ethics, Consequentialism, and Deontology.

To refresh our memory, in Chapter 3 we reviewed these theories:

- Virtue Ethics: The Good (character, constitution) conditions or produces the Right (choice, action).
- Consequentialism: The Good (end) justifies the Right (choice, action).
- Deontology: The Right (procedure) justifies the Good.

These three ethical theories, as Prof. Chidi Anagonye of *The Good Place* notes, are the basic ethical theories of the *W*estern tradition. The *Mahābhārata* depicts this as the morality of conventional times, in community, with others. All three are alike in giving the Good an important place in defining the Right. The dice game as a *metaphor* for conventional morality is used by the authors of the *Mahābhārata* to showcase its dangers. Prior to anyone playing the Game of Dice, the Pāṇḍavas were trying to live a life of conventional morality. They were trying to be good people who brought about good results and did good things. The Game of Dice was enticing as it was an opportunity to show off their virtue of courage, to aim for good outcomes (of winning), and for following the socially acceptable, good rules that constitute the game. Yet this model of conventional morality allows the Kauravas, the moral parasites, to direct hostility and violence toward the Pāṇḍavas. In effect, while the Pāṇḍavas were putting their energy into being conventionally moral, the Kauravas were harming them. And in case we think of this as a limited lesson, one could apply it to contemporary challenges too.

There are many systemic challenges, including colonialism, that face us today. Most people are likely conventionally moral. They object to colonialism, but they put all of their energy into conventional morality – of being good, hoping for a good outcome, and playing by good rules. That means that colonialism can still take advantage of them because the conventionally moral will not depart from the comfort of goodness to fight oppression.

As noted, there is a fourth ethical theory:

- Bhakti/Yoga: The Right conditions or produces the Good.

In Yoga, the Right is defined as a devotion to the ideal of the Right: Īśvara. Hence, one can understand the Right in general, and the right thing to do in specific cases, independently of the good. The good is a distant outcome of perfecting the Right. And hence, if one engages in Yoga, one doesn't have to get sucked into the trap of the moral parasite. The moral parasite uses goodness as bait. Good people, concerned with good outcomes and doing good things, are its victims. The Yogi can be free from colonial manipulation because they do not assume by virtue of their practice that they are participating in anything good. That allows them to discern what is bad, and to fight what is incompatible with their devotional practice.

ARJUNA'S LAMENT

The Game of Dice is a climax where the problem of Arjuna and the Pāṇḍavas comes to a head. It symbolizes their investment in conventional morality. It is hence no surprise that Arjuna falls back on the three ethical theories of conventional morality at the start of the *Bhagavad Gītā* to try to get out of fighting the inevitable war. Specifically, Arjuna provides three reasons against fighting:

- *Consequentialist Reason*: Fighting the conflict would kill loved ones on both sides. Even if he wins, the conflict will have wiped out his family (*Gītā* 1.34–36). This is like the Buddhist argument to minimize *dukkha* (suffering) – an end they call 'nirvāṇa'.
- *Virtue Theoretic Reason*: If the war is between good and evil, he is not evil like the Kauravas, yet fighting would make him no better than them (*Gītā* 1.38–39). Arjuna's reason here mirrors classical Jain Virtue Ethics: any action departs from the intrinsic goodness of the individual, as any action has some evil outcome – so one should just not get involved with anything.
- *Deontological Reason*: Conflict causes lawlessness, which is harmful to women and children (*Gītā* 1.41). War is primarily bad on this account as it does not respect laws.

A main problem with Arjuna's three reasons is that they assume that the problems they want to avoid have not already crystallized. If the problems already exist in advance of the war, then not fighting will not avoid them. And yet, Arjuna is theorizing *as though* these outcomes have yet to materialize. He is already pushed into a corner to fight, making him 'no better' than his opponents. He has already engaged in actions that produced lots of unhappiness. And he has already participated in the degradation of good social practices that compromise the safety of women. On Virtue Ethical, Consequentialist, and Deontological grounds, his life is already a failure.

*W*esterners, based on LAT, figure that social belonging and community are the answer to all our problems. This is a theme we see beginning with Plato and continuing in the tradition. What the *Mahābhārata* chronicles is how community is *where* we are oppressed and discriminated against. Arjuna is acting as though in choosing to fight he is giving up on the safety of community, when in reality, community is already a dangerous place for him. He is too busy trying to be conventionally moral to notice.

KṚṢṆA'S THREE RESPONSES

Kṛṣṇa provides two different sets of responses. Each set has three responses. The first set clearly addresses the concerns Arjuna raises. The second set is meant to get Arjuna away from thinking in terms of conventional morality of Virtue Ethics, Consequentialism, and Deontology.

Kṛṣṇa is Arjuna's childhood friend and relation. His first response then trades on their history: he begins by mocking Arjuna for his lack of valour and absence of courage in a time that requires decisive action. This is to appeal to a Virtue Ethical concern (*Gītā* 2.2–3, 2.33–37). He claims that paradise ensues for those who fight valiantly and die in battle – which is a Consequentialist concern (*Gītā* 2.36–37). Kṛṣṇa also claims that people are eternal, hence no one really destroys anyone else – which responds the Deontological worry that war corrupts good practice that protects individuals (*Gītā* 2.11–32). The last response is perhaps the most serious of the three, and Kṛṣṇa's subsequent arguments will go back to this.

Kṛṣṇa main responses that steer away from conventional morality are more radical: they do not simply respond to Arjuna's worry but rather provide positive guidance for how Arjuna can move forward. Specifically, Kṛṣṇa makes a case for two normative ethical theories and one metaethical theory.

First, Kṛṣṇa advances *Karma Yoga*. This is a version of Deontology. Deontology asks us to select, out of the many good things we can do, something that we have justifying reason to do: this is our duty. Kṛṣṇa extols the importance of *Karma Yoga* in terms of fidelity to duty, not any further outcome. He repeats: better one's own duty poorly performed than someone else's well performed (*Gītā* 2.38, 2.47, 18.47). Kṛṣṇa simply uses the term 'dharma' here for the thing that should be done.

What is our dharma? How do we determine that? Kṛṣṇa's wider discussion where he specifies *Karma Yoga* describes the thing to be done as our contribution to a world of diversity, given the particulars of our own life. He appeals to the sociological particulars of Arjuna's life, steeped in being a warrior, to fill in the details of what Arjuna should be doing. Kṛṣṇa claims that the right thing to do is specified by context-transcendent rules that take into account life capacities and situate us within a reciprocal arrangement of obligations and support (*Gītā* 12.5–13, 12.33–35). But we can certainly generalize from this discussion: a person's dharma is filled in by the sociological particulars of their life – their relationships to others and what they must do given these relationships. Hence, for instance, while I may be better at coaching a team of children who are not mine, on Kṛṣṇa's account, I should be taking care of my own children, even if I'm not as good at that.

It ought to go without saying that *Karma Yoga* is not the idea that we can barter our labour for free yoga classes – though I've seen this on sandwich boards at *āsana* schools. *Karma Yoga* is also not a yoga of service. It is primarily the yoga of perfecting one's sociological space. And one's dharma is not a mystery purpose that one has to figure out. It's what one needs to do given one's place in life.

The more exalted ethical practice that Kṛṣṇa argues for is *Bhakti Yoga*. This is basically the Yoga of the *Yoga Sūtra*. The essence of this practice is devotion to Īśvara (Kṛṣṇa here), and the good is just a distant outcome of the perfection of this practice. When Kṛṣṇa closes the *Gītā* with the famous line that Arjuna ought to *abandon all DHARMAS* – all moral principles, and rules – and come to him, and that he will release him from all faults (*Gītā* 18.66), Kṛṣṇa is in effect articulating Yoga as *Īśvara praṇidhāna* (devotion to Īśvara), which is the central practice of Yoga in the *Yoga Sūtra*. When we practise Yoga, as Patañjali teaches it, we are not following rules. It is our devotion to Īśvara and the practice of the essential traits of Sovereignty – unconservatism and self-governance – that produce the good outcome of the perfection of this practice. To engage in this is to abandon rules and to take on the responsibility of figuring out our life ourselves. But this is not a licentious practice. Whatever we do has to be part of this devotion to Īśvara, which means abandoning the idea we have figured it all out and affirming that more work (always) needs to be done. (In the *Yoga Sūtra*, Patañjali does provide the Eight Limbs, which are like rules. But they are *upāya*-s or remedies to practice. They are not the main practice: they are supports for the more basic practice of devotion.)

A third practice Kṛṣṇa prescribes is *Jñāna Yoga*. This is a metaethical practice of understanding. This involves the appreciation that ethical challenges and values are real. Kṛṣṇa as Īśvara claims that his role is to periodically reset the moral order (*Gītā* 4.7–8). But as the ideal of moral practice is the Right, it follows that there is no contradiction between the fact of evil and the ideal of the Right (*Gītā* 10.4–5). So a world and a practice governed by the ideal of the Right will have a lot of imperfection to contend with. This is an important point.

Theists who idealize a God who is all good have what is known as the *Problem of Evil*: how is it possible that there could be an all-Good God, who is responsible for the world, when there is so much evil in it? Here, the goodness of God seems incompatible with the evil of the world. But the Rightness of Īśvara is compatible with badness. Just as the Rightness of cleaning is compatible with a mess: just because there is a mess does not mean that cleaning is impossible or inappropriate. Just the opposite. So too is Rightness (cleaning) consistent with badness (a mess). Consider what is required to engage in a devotional practice toward the ideal of music. As one engages in this devotional practice to music, especially at the start, one will be bad at the practice of music. This does not mean that there is no such thing as an ideal of music that one ought to be devoted to. Rather, it is through this devotion that one can improve one's practice. Similarly, the reality of Īśvara as the Ideal of the Right is not inconsistent with the badness of people or the world. That's how things are when we have not made much progress in our devotional practice. But that does not entail that our practice was a mistake. We will only make improvements if we continue with practising. *Jñāna Yoga* involves appreciating all of this and an appreciation of ourselves as not essentially the same as the various natural features of the world, such as the three *guṇa*-s (we were introduced to these three qualities in Chapter 5). Rather, it is by devotion that we overcome external influence (*Gītā* 15.5).

In other classical sources of Yoga, such as the *Kaṭha Upaniṣad* or the *Yoga Sūtra*, we learn about a practice that can be defined independently of success criteria, which, if we perfect it, results in a good outcome. So, for instance, Yoga in the *Kaṭha Upaniṣad* is about coordinating the various aspects of one's life in service of the interest of the self (Sovereignty) and the good is the perfection of this practice. This is also front and centre in the *Bhagavad Gītā*. According to Kṛṣṇa, good things happen when people stick to their duty (*Gītā* 2.32). And in general, bad outcomes are avoided by paying attention to one's practice. But the important catch is that this is only possible if people are not acting for the sake of outcomes. To act for the sake of outcomes is to adopt Consequentialism. If we are Consequentialists and this motivates us to take up a practice, such as learning an instrument to play beautiful music, we will quit on day one or day two. Until we become proficient, we are bad at the practice. And no one is proficient at first. However, if we can stick with the practice, eventually we will bring about improvement in performance. But it is only possible to stick with it if we find meaning in the practice independently of the outcomes. So, too, with all practices of one's life. Bhakti – devotion to the Ideal of the practice of being a person, Īśvara – is essential to sustain such a practice: this leads to excellence in action that surmounts all challenges (*Gītā* 18.58).

CASTE

The *Bhagavad Gītā* and the *Mahābhārata* are not an exploration of what we should be doing in community with others. They are explorations of the challenges we face when community breaks down. Community breaks down because one part becomes obsessed with conventional morality. These are the 'good' people. The other part tries to take advantage of the conventionally moral. In reality, this relationship already constitutes a state of war, but it is not one that is obvious. The conventionally moral are the last to realize this. It is at this juncture that Yoga is the answer. We can practise Yoga at this point (and really at any point) because the practice of Yoga does not depend upon us being good. So even in bad times, when it's not easy or possible to be good, or when being good renders one a target of moral parasites, we can take up Yoga. Yoga is hence a practice of facing head on the problems of life. After Kṛṣṇa provides the three arguments of *Karma Yoga*, *Bhakti Yoga*, and *Jñāna Yoga* in the *Bhagavad Gītā*, he counsels the Pāṇḍavas (in subsequent chapters of the *Mahābhārata*) to lie, cheat, and steal in their war against the Kauravas. The Kauravas only have power because the Pāṇḍavas attempted to be conventionally good, rendering them easy targets for manipulation. Once the Pāṇḍavas stopped playing by conventional ethical rules, they were able to rid the world of these moral parasites. Many people tend to get confused as to how the Pāṇḍavas, guided by Kṛṣṇa, could lie, cheat, and steal and yet be counted as the good guys. But the confusion here is that to really meet the challenge, the Pāṇḍavas had to stop being the Good guys and start being the Right guys. Devotion to Īśvara makes us Right, and this allows us to get rid of evil. The devotee of Īśvara, unlike the moral parasite, is compassionate and cares about people on the whole. The moral parasite cares about no one but themselves.

As a template for action in life the *Bhagavad Gītā* brings to the fore that what we need to do to set things straight is to face problems head on and to give up on the conventional expectations of being good that keep us down. When we are worried about being good, we don't understand *how* evil works, because we won't allow ourselves to think that way. And the result is that we have no insight into the ways in which we are being targeted and manipulated. When we are worried about maximizing good outcomes, we don't engage in the activist practices we need to change the world we live in, for this involves bringing to the fore the unpleasantness of life. In fact, when we worry about bringing about good, we are easy targets for the bad man who points a gun to our head and says, 'If you don't kill two people, I will kill three.' Then, if we think it is our responsibility to bring about the best outcome (as Consequentialism dictates) under the circumstances, we become a tool of the bad man, and we will kill two. And when we are only focused on conventional good practices, we don't allow ourselves to innovate. We think of ethical behaviour as circumscribed by ostensible good practices.

It is hence somewhat paradoxical that caste ends up playing a role in Kṛṣṇa's discussions. The idea of 'caste' (*varṇa* in Sanskrit) is ancient in South Asia. Caste is so South Asian that there is no ancient community of people in South Asia who didn't have caste identities. Even the Buddha, as recorded in the *Pāli Canon*, who left conventional society, uses the term 'Brahmin' as a term of praise for well-informed people. Caste is also ancient in the West. For a clear argument for caste, we need to look to Plato's *Republic*. There he argues that the state is a reflection of the soul, and just as the soul has three parts (the reasonable, the active, and the appetitive) so too must there be three castes that comprise the state. And each caste is hence understood in terms of the role it plays in society.

Caste in South Asia allowed people a way to understand themselves independently of society. If one understands what one's caste is, then one has a way to appreciate what one could contribute to different societies. So people with caste identities could migrate to different communities.

The idea of caste receives lots of attention these days as it is the foundation for a lot of discrimination. In the Vedas, four castes are identified: the priests/intelligentsia/academics (*Brāhmaṇa*-s), the warrior/royal (*Kṣatriya*), those involved in commerce (*Vaiśya*), and manual labourers (*Śūdra*). And then, given this way of understanding how one can contribute to society, there is a fifth category of people: people with no caste identity, or the outcaste.

This is just a story, and the reality of caste is quite different. There weren't (and are not) just four castes and a fifth category of outcastes. There were hundreds if not thousands of castes. And still, to this day, the reality of caste is regional and diverse. Second, caste hierarchy is sustained by the literature written by Brahmins that celebrated themselves at the top. The British and other European colonizers deferred to this literature as information about South Asian society. But it's uncritical to accept that as a fact. The literary output of Brahmins that put them at the top of a list is in the first instance an example of self-serving propaganda. Certainly, many philosophies of ancient South Asia identified agents in a way that is distinct from their sociology. Hence, if you think that the self is different from facts like gender, sex, and species (as many South Asian philosophies do), it's hard to take the Brahmanical caste hierarchy that seriously.

When the British arrived, they attempted to 'understand' India by turning to Indigenous academics (Brahmins). (For a great review of this history, see Wilhelm Halbfass's *India and Europe.*) One result is that as the British created 'Hinduism', by labelling the entire South Asian tradition a religion, they also fabricated the idea of Hindu Law, which deferred to Brahmanical literature – especially caste purity manuals called the *dharmaśāstra*-s. And then, of course, just as South Asians start to believe they are Hindus, as a result of this, their understanding of caste also becomes less Indigenous. As my South Asian historiography professor (Narendra K. Wagle) pointed out to me some 25 years ago at the University of Toronto, while there is a hierarchy that puts the *Śūdra*-s at the bottom of the list, in the South of India, where most people were technically *Śūdra*-s, so too were many of the Tamil Kings and Emperors who were ostensibly at the top of the political structures in their regions. Colonialism had the effect of reifying Brahmanical stories about caste as though they were the Indigenous fact about caste.

The issue of caste when we look to Philosophy is even more complicated because philosophers do not agree as a rule, and many philosophies, especially Yoga, provide grounds for a nuanced criticism of caste.

To understand these criticisms, it's important to distinguish between caste as a description of our sociological status, and caste as a prescription. We could engage in the same kind of nuance with race. As a matter of description,

I am racialized as a South Asian: I'll be viewed as Brown in a racial hierarchy of White Supremacy. Acknowledging this does not justify or endorse the hierarchy: it rather reports the facts of how I'll be treated in this hierarchy. Then there is the idea that I ought to be treated as though I'm racially South Asian (whatever that entails). And clearly, I can acknowledge the descriptive racial identity as the foundations of a criticism of that identity. So I don't have to justify or endorse the identity just because I descriptively acknowledge it.

To acknowledge a descriptive caste identity is to be clear about the sociological particulars of one's ancestry and how that prepares one to contribute – economically – to society. In this sense, almost all of us have a caste identity. In reality, having highly educated parents helps students get an education and be successful at education. Having well-off, business-oriented parents helps children get set up and excel at business. Having parents who made their way in life via manual labour sets one up for more of the same. In our world today, we typically forbid explicit discrimination against someone on the basis of their sociological background. And yet, this doesn't mean that most societies have found a way to help people transcend the limits of their parents' knowledge and financial resources. And certainly, in the West, race, sex, and gender function as interpretive restrictions on people's opportunities in the way of discrimination. So while caste might be the grounds of discrimination (if we treat it as grounds for discrimination) that South Asians acknowledged caste descriptively does not entail that they had to endorse it prescriptively. And that they acknowledged it, like acknowledging racial identity, means that they could treat the descriptive grounds of caste as an opportunity to disrupt it.

Given this distinction between the descriptive and prescriptive approach to caste, the *Bhagavad Gītā* provides two different approaches to caste. One is descriptive but slightly subversive. The other is disruptive and anti-prescriptive.

The descriptive-subversive version is Kṛṣṇa's version of Deontology, *Karma Yoga*. In Kṛṣṇa's discussion of *Karma Yoga*, he describes it as the perfection of one's own dharma, and this is constrained by matters such as caste. The idea here is that all of us have some sociological context we are born into, which is a space that we can perfect, as a practice, that allows us to support ourselves and those who rely on us and thereby contribute to a universe of diversity. The dharma that we should perfect in *Karma Yoga* is one suited to one's nature (*Gītā* 18.41) and hence relatively easy to perfect. One's nature, *prakṛti*, is what comes from outside and influences one. One's nature is not one's essence as a person: it's just the external influences that define one's context. So *Karma Yoga* allows us a way to acknowledge these descriptive facts of our life as a way to make room for ourselves in a world of diversity. It is subversive in so far as the practice of *Karma Yoga* has to transform these external pressures into a recipe for personal success.

Bhakti Yoga, which is the Yoga of the *Yoga Sūtra*, and the *Kaṭha Upaniṣad*, is anti-prescriptive and disruptive of caste. That is because Yoga, original Yoga, is not about perfecting the space indicated to us by external pressure. It is about reclaiming our autonomy via devotion to Īśvara. When Kṛṣṇa speaks as Īśvara and tells Arjuna to abandon all 'dharmas', devote himself to Him, and He will liberate Arjuna from problematic activity (*Gītā* 18.66), he is describing what Yoga is like. As we are devoted to Sovereignty, we practise being sovereign via the essential traits of Sovereignty – unconservatism and self-governance. And that creates success. But this process is not about saving the space left to us by external pressure but rather clearing our space of personal intrusion. This is ethically and politically radical. Identity traits, such as race, sex, gender, species, religion, caste, are on the Yoga analysis *natural*: they are external to who we are as people. At our core, what it is to be a person is to be the kind of thing that has an interest in their unconservatism and self-governance. Hence, we could change superficial natural traits about ourselves – such as our sex or gender – and still be the same person! Today, this is important for us to reflect on, when in some parts of the world people react pathologically to others opting to choose their sexuality, gender, or sex. Really, there could be nothing more Yogic than actually choosing how to express one's personhood.

CHAPTER 6 REFLECTIONS

- What is conventional morality?
- How is conventional morality definitive of the West?
- What do the *Mahābhārata* and the *Bhagavad Gītā* teach us about conventional morality?
- *Karma Yoga* is a form of Deontology. How is it like *Bhakti Yoga*? How is it different?

» *Ahiṃsā* is often depicted as not breaking things. How is the Yoga approach to *ahiṃsā* different from ordinary notions?

» Why do we find the model of the chariot from the *Upaniṣads* being used in the *Bhagavad Gītā*?

» When Yoga disrupts conventional ethical expectations, how is this practice different from the ethical malfeasance of moral parasites?

» What is Yoga/Bhakti, and how does it differ from conventional ethical theories?

» How can small 'y' yoga practice embody the disruption of Bhakti/Yoga?

» How can *Karma Yoga* be subversive? How is *Bhakti Yoga* disruptive?

CHAPTER 7

'MODERN YOGA' AND COLONIAL TRAUMA

How came it that English supremacy was established in India? ... Such a country and such a society, were they not the predestined prey of conquest? ... India, then, could not escape the fate of being conquered, and the whole of her past history, if it be anything, is the history of the successive conquests she has undergone. Indian society has no history at all – at least no known history. What we call its history, is but the history of the successive intruders who founded their empires on the passive basis of that unresisting and unchanging society.

The question, therefore, is not whether the English had a right to conquer India, but whether we are to prefer India conquered by the Turk, by the Persian, by the Russian, to India conquered by the Briton. England has to fulfill a double mission in India: one destructive, the other regenerating – the annihilation of old Asiatic society, and the laying of the material foundations of Western society in Asia. Arabs, Turks, Tartars, Moguls, who had successively overrun India, soon became Hinduized, the barbarian conquerors being, by an eternal law of history, conquered themselves by the superior civilization of their subjects.

The British were the first conquerors superior, and, therefore, inaccessible to Hindu civilization... The day is not far distant when, by a combination of railways and steam vessels, the distance between England and India, measured by time, will be shortened to eight days, and when that once fabulous country will thus be actually annexed to the Western World.

Marx and Engels (1853)[1]

INTRODUCTION

Western colonialism operates by treating the very tradition that brings us White Supremacy and colonialism *as* our source of knowledge on moral and political matters, as well as history. Whether they are conscious of it or not, Western academics usually employ major moral and political doctrines from the Western tradition as a kind of backdrop that informs how they are to think about the colonized peoples and traditions they cover. In the West there are two extremes that tend to dominate. Toward the Conservative side, we have Liberalism. (It is remarkable that in the US this is considered a centre-left position! The more 'conservative' positions here and in other Western countries are some form of White nationalism – though that is not so far off from Liberalism.) And toward the purportedly revolutionary side, we have Marxism.

Perhaps the most influential Liberal is John Stuart Mill. Mill's day job was with the British East India Company. He was a professional colonizer. He is famous for defending Liberalism in *On Liberty*. There he argues that everyone should be free to experiment (*tapas*) and determine their own conception of the good (*svādhyāya*). What is rarely noted, because most do not appreciate South Asian moral philosophy, is that Mill appropriated Yoga. In Yoga, experimentation (*tapas*) and determining one's own values (*svādhyāya*) produce no extra outcome: they are a procedural reclaiming of one's own autonomy and part of one's Devotion to Sovereignty. Hence, the end of Yoga is called *kaivalya* – isolation (YS IV.34). Moral and political activism is based on this radical respect for every individual's autonomy as a function of Īśvara, the procedural ideal of the Right. And this might involve taking sides on behalf of people, and against the moral parasite. For Mill, as a Utilitarian, the point of this appropriation of Yoga is to maximize happiness. This entails nothing about the distribution of happiness and hence it is consistent with conservatism and oppression. One can, by this scheme, produce 100 units of happiness, which go to just one out of 100 people. Or, one could have a scheme where every one of 100 people gets just one unit of happiness. Utilitarianism as a form of Consequentialism cannot distinguish between these outcomes as they are the same outcome: 100 units of happiness. And so, perhaps unsurprisingly, we find Mill explicitly claiming that the freedoms he defends are not for racially immature people like South Asians, who would be so lucky as to find themselves an Akbar – one of India's famous Muslim Emperors.

Mill is also famous for a plea to protect minorities against the 'tyranny of the majority'. In *W*estern societies, people from colonized traditions often seem to be the minority. What is rarely noted is that in Mill's case, *he*, as the British colonizer, was the actual minority, colonizing South Asia. And in fact, White people the world over are a racial minority if the options are just two: being White, and not being White. Minority rights are often seen in the *W*est as a benevolent approach to protecting individuals in society. But the historical origins of this idea are menacing. And if we want to see modern evidence of its racist origins, we need only consider the racist 'replacement theory' bandied about by the Far Right in the *W*est who are fearful of being replaced by Black and Brown people. It is a fear driven by the demographic shift in the US, where White people are headed to being a minority. According to Yoga, injustice is really a function of failing to treat individuals as individuals, with their own needs and requirements. Oppression shown to anyone – White, Black, Trans, Bhūma Devī (the Earth), Dog, or Pig – is wrong because persons share an interest in their own Īśvara (their own *tapas* and *svādhyāya*), and oppression denies our shared interests. This interest is not reducible to how we look, or how we behave, but to what we require to thrive. Every person thrives given a healthy relationship to their past (unconservatism/*tapas*) and a self-determination of the values that will govern their future (self-governance/*svādhyāya*). The reduction of personhood to some empirical description or presentation of a person (such as their sex, species, or pigment) is wrong, as it simply misses what is important about being a person. Thinking about injustice as the bullying of the minority by the majority fails to explain *why* this is wrong, but it also provides cover for the White Supremacist and the colonizer who is the ultimate minority. Globally, the bullying of the majority by the minority (*W*estern colonialism) is a bigger threat but wrong for the same reason: it undermines people's *kaivalya*. It is hence no surprise that actual social justice and activism derives not from the White Supremacy of Mill but the Yoga of Patañjali, as noted in Chapters 1 and 4.

Some sickened by Liberalism's failure to respond to the challenges of colonized people turn to Marx and Engels, progenitors of Marxism. But this is absurd too. The main problem with South Asia is that it has been colonized for centuries, and that colonizers, like Marx and Engels, think that it is fitting that South Asia was colonized.

Marx is famous for a very important criticism of Capitalism. Capitalism is the economic system defined by two classes: the worker and the capitalist. The capitalist has private wealth to invest in the production of goods that they sell, and the workers (paid by the capitalist) just get a pay cheque for their time: they don't own what they make, nor are they fully compensated for the value they create. The capitalist rather keeps this surplus value (gross income minus the cost of running a business) as their own 'capital' to be invested again. Marx points out that this is indeed exploitative: because the worker does not own the means of production, they are deprived of the wealth they create. But what does this have to do with the problems of South Asia? The problems of South Asia are the problems of colonialism. But Marx and his partner in writing, Engels, take this to be the Indigenous way of South Asians. They are hence not friends of South Asians. There are some structural similarities between the colonizer and the capitalist and the worker and the colonized. But to conflate them is to fail to appreciate what colonialism is. It's not just being forced to take a low-paying job to make ends meet, which is the plight of the worker under Capitalism. Colonialism is a total annihilation of the personhood of the colonized in terms of the interpretive outlook of the colonizer. But certainly, the combination of Capitalism and Imperialism can be devastating. As Profs. Utsa Patnaik and Prabhat Patnaik note,[2] Britain managed to drain wealth from India (of the order of $45 trillion) by taxing Indians and then buying products from Indians with their own money. Then, further, the British made others who wanted to buy Indian goods purchase them from the British. This allowed the British to drain wealth from India as capital. And this scheme is possible even as Indians themselves owned the means of production! This is also a problem for Britain today, where many people act and choose as though they are this same colonial power of the past, and not a very small country on the border of a larger economic unit. To quote the Sex Pistols: England is dreaming.

What is notable about Marx and Engels' view is that as *W*estern colonizers, they revile and treat the colonized culture as a fixed entity, independent of colonization. Colonization does not alter or change the colonized for the worst, on this view. If anything (according to Marx and Engels), the real problem is that the culture of South Asia is *too* resilient and ends up swallowing up the colonizer. According to them, we need something more White Supremacist: something that will transform the colonized into something better, less problematic, and more like European society. In this description of South Asians, Marx and Engels betray two competing narratives of South Asia: (1) the problems of South Asia are a result of the Indigenous tradition and not a function of colonialism, and (2) there is no precolonial history of South Asia: it's just colonialism all the way back. South Asians are fit for colonization, in their view, as it's just their way of life.

In most ways, the study of South Asia, including Yoga Studies, has not moved passed the White Supremacy of Marx and Engels.

In South Asian Studies and Religious Studies, everyone knows that South Asian religious identity, like being Hindu, is created under British colonialism. And yet, these categories are read backwards into the history of South Asia as though there is no precolonial history to India: it's just colonialism all the way back. Worse, (1) the parts of the tradition that many reject, like prescriptive views on caste, rejected by Yoga/Bhakti, get pegged as defining features of Hinduism, which is the colonial word for Indigenous South Asian religion, whatever that is. In this way, the problems of Hinduism are Indigenous (caste). And yet (2) there is no precolonial history. Whatever is known under colonialism as defining Hinduism is just the way it's always been. And hence academics talk about 'Hindu Law'. This includes prescriptive views on caste, as though that defines Hinduism, precolonially, before the religion was invented.

Yoga Studies has its own version of Marx and Engels' confusion, which at once identifies yoga in terms of its colonial manifestations and treats it as though there is no prehistory to colonialism: it's colonial yoga all the way back. Everyone in Yoga Studies knows about 'modern yoga'. This is Yoga that was being taught under British colonialism. As noted in Chapter 2, modern yoga today is completely *WAC*-ky: it requires pedagogies and organizational structures defended in Plato's *Republic* – which forms the basis for lineages as the primary pedagogical tool – and absent from any ancient text of Yoga philosophy. (1) Yet the problematic nature of modern yoga, even though it began under colonialism, is treated as Indigenous. And yet (2) there is no discussion of precolonial Yoga – actual Yoga – without using 'modern yoga' as the model. To get away from lineages, Yoga Studies writers talk about 'post-lineage' yoga. So in this way, the *WAC*-ky yoga of lineages, colonial as it is, problematic as it is, is treated as the way it's always been.

What is going on here, with Marx and Engels and all who follow suit, is interpretation. Interpretation leads us to use beliefs created by colonialism (a political process itself created by interpretation) as our explanation of the past. And then, the colonized are viewed timelessly as they are under colonization, and there is never any precolonial past: it's colonialism all the way back. Politically, we can think about the challenge of breaking with this. It's not about interpreting the world according to a different set of facts. It's about giving up on interpretation altogether to explicate the options. And this shows that the options we have now are different from the precolonial options. And the options that are familiar to us under colonialism, like 'modern yoga', are a fabrication of colonialism. Identifying them as Yoga is a mistake with political implications.

EARLY COLONIAL SOUTH ASIA

'Modern yoga', or 'modern postural yoga', is the yoga we do in a yoga school or at some specific time of the day set aside for our *āsana* practice. And importantly, 'modern yoga' is about treating that very delimited practice as the paradigm case of yoga – and not just one way to practise yoga. Those who are more reflective practitioners of 'modern yoga' spend time thinking about how those practices, undertaken in very delimited contexts, could carry benefits in other areas of life. From here we get the idea that yoga practice is primarily something that happens 'on the mat' and then there is a derivative practice that is '*off* the mat'. In actual Yoga, there's no mat. But the mat – the designated space for the practice of yoga – is centrally important to 'modern yoga'.

This approach to Yoga is associated with modern South Indian teacher, Tirumalai Krishnamacharya (1888–1989) who taught Indra Devi (1899–2002), K. Pattabhi Jois who went on to be the founder of *Ashtanga Yoga* (1915–2009), B. K. S. Iyengar who created *Iyengar Yoga* (1918–2014), T. K. V. Desikachar (1938–2016), Srivatsa Ramaswami (born 1939), and A. G. Mohan (born 1945). Krishnamacharya's influence cannot be underestimated. Most people the world over today practise some form of small 'y' yoga that originates from some teacher who either studied with Krishnamacharya or is in a lineage of teachers going back to Krishnamacharya. There are certainly other origins of postural yoga. Mark Singleton in his widely read *Yoga Body*[3] claims that what we think of as this Indian practice of yoga is a repackaging of gymnastic trends popular in Europe at the time of Krishnamacharya. In the stronger version of the claim from Singleton's book, South Asians lacked any history of *āsana* practice and that was an innovation brought on by Western influence.

First off, there is certainly a history that predates European colonialism of yoga *āsana* practice. We find it in many earlier texts, including the one we shall examine in the next section. The idea that this was purely an adoption of Western gymnastic practices is a remarkably false claim.

But given an explicatory appreciation of Yoga as foundationally a practice of devotion to Īśvara, which consists in practising the essential traits of Sovereignty, namely *tapas* (unconservatism) and *svādhyāya* (self-governance), anything can be small 'y' yoga if it is a way to practise Yoga. And hence the cultural origins of particular postures or activities do not count against it being Yoga, nor do they show that Yoga is a novel invention inspired by Europeans. Singleton's point about the cultural origins of some small 'y' practices is perhaps interesting but ultimately unimportant. What makes something Yoga is not the cultural origins of the practice but whether it is a way to practise capital 'Y' Yoga. If one is practising Yoga, then anything one does is a way to practise Yoga.

What accounts for the gulf that separates an understanding of Yoga and the elevation of small 'y' practices to the paradigm cases of yoga and the jettisoning of Yoga? How did it ever come to pass that people have largely got it backwards? To not have it backwards is to begin with Yoga and then decide to practise something as small 'y' yoga. Instead, some story about small 'y' yoga has taken over, and people are largely confused about how there could have been any precolonial Yoga. The answer is bound up with *W*estern colonialism.

This requires first some appreciation of Indian history. Historically, many people have fled to South Asia and what we today call 'India' as refugees or in search of safe residence. Ancient groups that arrived on South Asian soil include Christians, one of the oldest groups of Jews known as the 'Bene Israel' who according to their account have been in India for nearly two millennia, and Zoroastrians who fled Persia as it was being Islamicized. Many of these groups brought with them the idea of religious identity, which as noted was created by the Romans to normalize the subjugation of colonized traditions in *W*estern empire. The influx of people with these identities in South Asia did not alter much as they did not come as colonizers. However, with the beginning of Islamic conquests, such as the Delhi Sultanate (1206–1526 CE), things changed. For political institutions brought with them ideas of *W*estern colonialism, namely religion, as part of their understanding of state structure and social order. This was the start of *W*estern colonialism in South Asia. And this was in many ways violent.

In ancient times in South Asia, it's very hard to find any example of rulers who expected the ruled to convert to their outlook. Hence, martyrdom is quite an unheard of phenomenon in ancient South Asia. The idea that one needs to die for one's beliefs would have made no sense to ancient South Asians.

One might die while fighting the right fight (as Kṛṣṇa counsels Arjuna) but then what is at stake is not a belief system but personal autonomy, independence, and Sovereignty. Unlike in the *West*, which begins with the murder of Socrates, followed by the crucifixion of Jesus, and a seemingly endless list of political persecutions of intellectuals, that didn't happen in ancient South Asia. That is because South Asia was not, originally, a place of interpretation (explanation in terms of belief). That is because South Asia lacked the LAT that conflates what we would say (typically what we believe) with what we can think. And hence, South Asians could separate thinking from believing. And hence, as a matter of public policy, no one seemed to think that we had to share the same beliefs to get on with each other in part because no one really took belief seriously. In fact, as I point out in my chapter on logic in my book *Hinduism: A Contemporary Philosophical Investigation* (2018), the famous myth of the Churning of the Milk Ocean not only presents us with a useful model for logic but also indicates how historical South Asians thought about dissent.

The story begins with the gods (devas) worrying about reputational risk. They head over to Viṣṇu who hatches a plan: they have to enlist the cooperation of their demonic cousins to churn the Milk Ocean to gain the nectar of immortality; once they consume it, they won't have to worry about reputational risk. The demonic cousins want the nectar too, so they agree to the scheme. The agitator, a mountain that churns the ocean, rests on Viṣṇu in a specific form: the turtle – an animal that withdraws its senses and hence symbolizes *Pratyāhāra*. The rope of this tug of war between the demons and the gods that is pushed and pulled hence moves the agitator that rests on *Pratyāhāra*. And this means that the churning is an exercise of reason, as reason is about understanding the force of positions, but on the basis of *Pratyāhāra* – the nonempirical. In churning, each side understands the force of the other side, but also that their perspective is a completely contingent feature of *where they are* and not about *who they are*. Logical understanding is largely about appreciating the force of some perspective without having to agree! This is the push and pull of that churning exercise.

There are lots of loops and turns in the story. At one point in the process, the poison of a sense of futility is emitted and they have to enlist the help of Śiva the destroyer to get rid of it: he swallows it but his consort, Śakti, stops it at his throat (thus he becomes Nīla-kaṇṭha, the Blue-throated). He gets rid of the problem by being silent about it. Everyone resumes the churning.

Eventually, the nectar emerges: the demons try to steal it for themselves. Viṣṇu comes back as Mohinī, the beautiful enchantress, who the demons deputize to distribute the nectar: she only gives it to the gods. (Incidentally, anyone curious about the implications of *tapas* and Yoga for issues of sex and gender need look no further than Viṣṇu, *tapas*, choosing gender and sex as means of personal expression.) The churning process of pulling symbolizes the task of understanding the force of the perspective you do not agree to or give in to. And the gods, unlike the demons, are willing to live indefinitely with those they disagree with. And so the moral of the story is that what it is to be venerable for all of eternity is to be willing to get along with those you disagree with. This is the way to overcome reputational risk! This is a completely Indigenous South Asian way of modelling proper public behaviour. It is Secularism_1: everyone is welcome to participate in logical disagreement. But the logical disagreement is not about who you are. Rather, it is about the force of third-party perspectives you do not have to assent to. This means, ultimately, we can respect each other without having to define each other in terms of our contingent perspectives.

As a story of Philosophy, this myth represents what South Asians valued in earlier times. They were open to philosophical dissent and discussion. No one had to be part of social convention: they could decide to operate on the boundaries of society like the Buddha as a *śramaṇa*. And moreover, this kind of philosophical independence that was the basis for public disagreement was valued as an important part of the world. And, importantly, there was no religion: just philosophical disagreement on topics like dharma. We know this because when we explicate the history of South Asian thought, we find moral disagreements on dharma. The story is also Yogic. Everyone involved is engaged in the *tapas* of understanding the force of others' positions and the *svādhyāya* of owning their choices that inform their activity. And everyone is in effect devoted to Īśvara, Sovereignty, as they desire that nectar of immortality.

But with the rise of Western colonialism in South Asia, there is a departure from this idea that public interaction is about disagreement. The South Asian tradition moves increasingly to the standard Western model of top-down, doctrinal enforcement. This is solidified by the British who tell South Asians who are not Muslims that they are Hindus. Colonizers create and foster ideas of Hinduism (Indianism) not as a Secular_1 disagreement on everything (as was the case historically) but in terms of shared doctrines and outlooks. In

Chapter 2, we reviewed how the colonial transmission of LAT led to the creation of a 'Muslim' (Urdu) and 'Hindu' (Hindi) language out of the same spoken language (Hindustani) and that these in turn formed the *Western* foundations for the Secularism$_2$ Pakistan and India.

In this process of *Westernization*, those who are viewed as not willing to convert or endorse the 'official' position are treated as worthy of violence, and not worthy of moral consideration. What the earlier manifestation of this process of *Western* (Islamic) colonization managed to do was to make the idea of martyrdom an Indigenous South Asian idea when it wasn't before. The martyrdom of Sikh gurus, starting with Guru Arjan (1563–1606 CE) by the Muslim Moghul emperor, Jahangir (1569–1627 CE), is a great example. Arjan is reported to have been imprisoned and tortured to force him to renounce Sikhism. He refused and as a result he was martyred. Sikhism was a new South Asian religion created in Panjab by Guru Nanak (1469–1539 CE), who was born in the Delhi Sultanate. If it was like precolonial South Asian positions, it would have had no awareness of martyrdom – or religion. But as a result of the Sikh experience with Islamic rulers, the martyr (*śahīd*) is now part of a tradition created in South Asia.[4]

There are many ways in which the history of Islamic colonization is hard to reduce to a single description. Some rulers were despotic and destructive. Others like Akbar – who Mill thinks should rule South Asians – were famed for stressing the importance of religious pluralism and an openness to learning from South Asians. The praise he receives however is a function of a very low bar: he's credited, for instance, with not destroying temples. Sure, he was nicer than others who held his job. But what standard *Western* retellings of this colonial history try to hide is that the seemingly benign expressions of the Secuarlism$_2$ of the *West*, complete with religious identity as a way of understanding the non-*Western* options, was *Western* colonialism succeeding. Instead of the Indigenous Secularism$_1$ of South Asia, *Western* narratives prefer the idea of religious pluralism of Secularism$_2$. And to be explicit, Secularism$_2$ is the oldest form of White Supremacy, as it treats the *Western* tradition as the default content of public secular life everywhere and Indigenous BIPOC traditions, like Secularism$_1$, as something that has to be banished from the secular as it is religious. As I have pointed out in my work, the intolerance to diversity we increasingly see in South Asia is a direct result of banishing its history of open philosophical dissent as a specific religion (Hinduism) that has no place in the secular state – a religion that is then not understood in terms of its precolonial past but in terms of some supposed shared perspective that is created under colonialism. And once Secularism_2 sets in, South Asians lose an ancestral connection to their ancient Secularism_1 past and understand themselves in terms of their marginalization under Secularism_2. I have been surprised that scholars of South Asian religion do not appreciate how colonialism has simultaneously undermined South Asian capacity for engaging diversity but also created a monster, namely xenophobic religious identity. I have been surprised that these authors do not observe that: if we were to go fully Indigenous in South Asia, and anticolonial, we would have to get rid of religious identity all together and reclaim the ancient practice of doing Philosophy out in the open. It might be this realization that their way of studying South Asia depends upon colonial concepts of religion that stops them from doing decolonial scholarship. But decolonial scholarship is historical. Colonial 'scholarship' reapplies categories created by colonialism as interpretive explanations of what happened before these colonial innovations. It's not scholarship: it's just more colonialism.[5]

I have been around South Asianists, Indologists, and their modern offspring, Yoga Studies authors, for a long time. And what I have observed is that these academic writers are loath to talk about Islamic colonization. The Liberal Millians among them perceive such discussion as a discrimination against the minority. This means that the majority of South Asians can never complain about any version of colonization, including the European version, as this would be bullying the minority. And the Marxists think that colonization is just the way South Asians live and it is intrinsic to their history – on this view, there really is no noticeable difference between Islamic conquest and the history of South Asia, as (falsely) they think it's just always been that way. For Marxists, it's all just more religious strife. The not-so 'sub' text of these explanations is a White Supremacy that treats the problems of South Asia not as a function of colonization but the failure of South Asians to be more like White people, especially the British. But this is a problem, for in pretending that this was a nonevent, academic authors miss the origins of *Western* colonialism in South Asia and then *do not* track the changes that happened in the South Asian tradition as a function of that colonization. They rather treat these changes as though they are fully Indigenous.

One fear that I'm sure many colonial academic authors have is that they do not want to appear to be proponents of the Hindu Right, when the talking points of the Hindu Right frequently involve criticizing *Western* intrusion.

But we don't have to fall for this poor reasoning. Explication reveals that the Hindu Right is also not an Indigenous position but a continuation of Western colonialism based on linguistic and religious identity bequeathed by British colonizers.

Poorly reasoned, it seems like criticizing Islamic colonizers is tantamount to criticizing all Muslims. But that's not true. Criticizing British colonizers is not the same as criticizing all British people. As a Canadian, I can criticize my Canadian colonial ancestors without thinking that I'm guilty of the same crime. Indeed, the possibilities of my own decolonial activity depend upon my ability to distinguish between the choices colonizing Canadians made and the ones I can make. This decision to avoid discussion of the colonial choices of our ancestors because it makes us uncomfortable is actually motivating laws in the US that aim to ban the discussion of racism if it makes White people feel bad (such as Florida's 2022 Senate Bill 148 or Texas's House Bill 3979 signed into law). In the US these discussions are punctuated by paranoia about 'critical race theory' being taught in kindergarten – and it never was, as critical race theory is a legal theory of interest to the study of Law. But what we find in the discussion of South Asia is a self-censorship about colonialism because it might make people feel bad.

Our Yogic analysis frames the problem of Western colonization in terms of a loss of skills for public diversity. As Secularism$_2$ took over, the explicatory practices of Secularism$_1$ disappeared. So people stopped being able to get along with others by disagreeing. Increasingly, they were comfortable only with those who agreed with them or shared their perspective, and they hid away from public dissent. And all the while, public space in South Asia was increasingly dangerous owing to waves of conquests. And so, the problem was not that Muslims showed up in South Asia. It was that the interpretive practices of the West started to take over. And here too, we can tell the problem is not some part of Western culture showing up. It's *interpretation* that shows up as a colonial frame in South Asia that is the problem. When we interpret, we can only appreciate what we believe, and anything that deviates seems like a threat to our outlook, which we confuse with ourselves. So interpretation creates violence and public uncertainty. The martyrdom of Sikh gurus is one dramatic example of this. The ordinary violence that ordinary South Asians experienced as a result of this colonization is another.

And finally, without appreciating this history, we cannot appreciate this weird thing called 'modern yoga'.

THE *HAṬHA YOGA PRADĪPIKĀ*

Against the backdrop of this radical social change in South Asia occasioned by the start of Western colonialism in 1206 CE, we find the famous *Haṭha Yoga Pradīpikā* by Svātmārāma (written circa 1400 CE). The *Haṭha Yoga Pradīpikā* is an example of what I call *applied yoga* texts. Applied yoga texts focus on small 'y' yoga. But they also tend to specify limbs of yoga, and the limbs often diverge from each other and the earlier list we find in Patañjali's *Yoga Sūtra*. A famous earlier *applied yoga text* is the *Yoga Yājñavalkya*, which likely was authored around the beginning of the first millennium CE.

The *Haṭha Yoga Pradīpikā*, while similar to other texts in being an applied yoga text, departs from the *Yoga Sūtra* and earlier sources of Yoga philosophy in many ways. First, whereas we find Viṣṇu either explicitly mentioned or implicitly celebrated (as *tapas*, with the three *kriyā*-s) in earlier Yoga philosophy texts, this text begins by praising Ādinātha, which is a title for Śiva. In South Asian philosophy, Śiva is associated with Consequentialist theories, whether Kāśmīra Śaivism, or Nyāya and Vaiśeṣika. The Nath tradition that treats this text as an important source is also explicitly a Śaiva tradition. While Western interpretation treats talk of deities as a mysterious irrelevance, when we explicate the history of South Asia we see that South Asians celebrated their ideals in art and literature. Śiva is classically depicted as the ideal experiencer, and his partner, Śakti, is his range of experiences. Whereas Viṣṇu, as *tapas*, is a deity depicted as actively engaging with others in public, Śiva is classically depicted either in lotus position with his eyes close or as Naṭarāja, the Lord of Dance, ushering the destruction of the universe. He is happy when he is not woken up and is reported to spew fire from his third eye at anyone who disturbs his meditation. Śiva is benign in this state, but terrible (Rudra) when he is bothered.

While knowledge of this practice of yoga is generally confused (HYP I.3) Svātmārāma describes the lineage of teachers that he learned it from (HYP I.4). Those who perfected this practice are free to roam about the universe (HYP I.5). The nomenclature of calling the prescribed form of small 'y' yoga practice '*haṭha*' is paradoxical. According to the *Monier-Williams Sanskrit-English Dictionary*, it means 'forceful', 'violent', 'oppressive', 'going in the rear of the enemy'. Yet it is described as something one does in retreat. It is a protection from the heat of *tapas*: for those who perfect the practice it is like assuming the abilities of the tortoise who withdraws its senses (HYP I.6). The practice, however, must be kept secret in order for it to yield powers

(HYP I.7). It must be practised inside a cottage (*maṭha*) in a virtuous, well-ruled kingdom, which is free from disturbances (HYP I.12). The practice that is to be done is the practice taught by the human teacher and it is by their grace that channels of internal power, *kuṇḍalinī*, are awakened in the student (HYP III.2). Indeed, real advance in practice is to be gained by the teacher's instruction, and not via the study of various texts (HYP III.78). The real Īśvara is actually the human guru, themselves appropriately trained by a guru, who imparts this knowledge to the student – or the human guru is to be understood as the visible manifestation of Īśvara (HYP III.129).

The entire picture of what yoga is in this text is a Consequentialist retelling of Yoga. In Yoga our project is regaining one's own autonomy (*kaivalya*) in a world with others. Autonomy itself only makes sense if there are others that one is separate from, and so, perhaps paradoxically, *kaivalya* is a social idea. Our autonomy is not anything extra: it's just us without the issues or the manipulation. It's what we already have, but it's trampled on by external influence (*prakṛti*). When we attain it, via an ethical transformation that gets rid of interpretation, we realize the ways in which others are not in states of autonomy but also that our past and future are real. But that is a knowledge we have because we can explicate ourselves and others, relative to the past and the future (as discussed in *Yoga Sūtra*, Book 4). Here, in the *Haṭha Yoga Pradīpikā*, small 'y' yoga is retooled as the means of various powers. In the *Yoga Sūtra*, powers are acknowledged as an outcome of the practice of Yoga, but they are also critically assessed as a distraction (YS III.38). We are safe so long as we are engaging powers not as a means to an end but as part of our practice of reclaiming our autonomy. Here, in the *Haṭha Yoga Pradīpikā* the powers are a means to an end: one's liberation, conceptualized (ironically) as a free movement after death (HYP I.5–9). And specifically, to get this work going, one has to be enthusiastic, persevere, engage in discrimination, have unshakable faith and courage, *and* avoid the company of people who are unsuitable (HYP I.15). This latter direction is most telling. In original Yoga, there is no basis for avoiding 'common' or 'unsuitable' people. Indeed, the myth of the Churning of the Milk Ocean that brings together classical Yogic practices of *tapas* (the pulling) and *svādhyāya* (owning one's own position) is a devotional exercise to Sovereignty (the nectar) we need the nonyogic demons to practise with.

Our actual Yoga practice is what we do with others, who may not be practising at all. Yoga is not a group project. It's our own work to be a person in the company of other people. But for the *Haṭha Yoga Pradīpikā*, yoga is something one does indoors, in a specific place, under the tutelage of a human teacher, in a gentrified part of the world, and is very different from what one would engage in outside, with ordinary, undesirable, or common people. Sound familiar? This is 'modern yoga'. This is the yoga that is dependent upon human tutelage and tied to specific places. The practice of yoga as something that one does on the mat, primarily, and then metaphorically *off the mat* is a modern extension of this vision of yoga.

If we interpret, we use our beliefs about yoga to explain the past of yoga, and then we cannot understand the past as anything different from the presently derived beliefs we use to explain it. So in this way, the past is inaccessible to us. If we explicate, we can see a massive, seismic, shift from original, early, precolonial Yoga to the cowering in a corner of the *Haṭha Yoga Pradīpikā*. Original Yoga is its own basic ethical theory: its own view on *THE RIGHT OR THE GOOD*. Specifically, it is the idea that by being devoted to the Right – to the ideal of the Right – we create a practice that is personal, and the perfection of that practice is the good. There's no extra outcome and nothing outside of ourselves to achieve. Our completion of the practice is just the reclamation of our agency. This is radically decolonial and anti-oppressive. In the *Haṭha Yoga Pradīpikā*, we see a pronounced shift to Consequentialism. The practices of small 'y' yoga are to be undertaken for the end they bring about. And it is because of this promise of the end that we must obey our human guru who is legitimized by who they in turn studied with but also the powers they have, but powers that are not really visible outside of the closed place of practice. This practice leaves colonialism as it is and looks instead for a safe space to practise esoteric powers that, objectively, disappear the moment we step out of the place of practice.

YOGA IN HIDING?

One response I've heard from students in light of these observations about the correlation between Islamic colonization in South Asia and the hiding, secretive practice outlined in the *Haṭha Yoga Pradīpikā* is that these modifications to yoga were necessary to survive given the external oppression and violence of colonization. And indeed, this trend to conceive of pedagogy as a transmission of doctrine from teacher to student lineages as the anchor of practices that are internal to groups becomes more and more of a thing after the rise of Western colonization. And this move to human-lineages is different from the succession of teachers from precolonial traditions. In the precolonial form, the celebrated teachers are inspirations for what our own practice could look like. These teachers, such as the child Yogi, Namāḻvār, or the young woman, Āṇḍāḷ, who determined her own sexuality and choice of partner, *lived life on their own terms*. That's why they are an inspiration to us – from afar with no direct social contact. In the colonial version of 'yoga', the human-lineage is treated as *the chief* pedagogical means of learning yoga, and this is only real in actual social interaction – behind closed doors. And whereas, before, the primary teacher was the abstraction, Īśvara, which we had to take responsibility for by being devoted to it (which means we had to make the challenge of being sovereign our own problem), this colonized version of 'yoga' makes it the human teachers' problem to *learn us good*. In colonized yoga, we live life on our teacher's terms. But perhaps this is exactly the point of the sympathizer: we need this human-lineage to pass along the knowledge in colonial contexts because colonialism allows nothing else.

This later claim makes no sense. If learning about Yoga is really about our own devotion to Īśvara, then it wouldn't matter what the context is. And indeed, under colonialism there is even a greater need for a public devotion to Īśvara, for colonialism tries to deprive us of Sovereignty, and our own public devotion to Īśvara is the way to regain our autonomy: this is the war of the *Gītā*. 'Modern yoga' is not a way to make Yoga survive under colonialism. It's a relabelling of colonial, trauma-based behaviour as yoga. It is the egotism of colonization haunted by the name of the previous, free practice of Yoga. The reason that Consequentialism plays such a prominent role in this trauma-based behaviour is that egotism sets this up as the primary way to function. When we identify with an outlook, and thereby construct a false sense of self that is egotism, our agency is then deployed to normalize this sense of self. As the outlook is the end, our agency is seen purely as a means to this end. It has no intrinsic value any more and is only valued as far as it protects and restores the outlook and whatever it values or desires. Yet once this ego is in charge, it wants the comfort of external validation (the good human teacher who will learn you good) and good rules to practise. Conventional morality (good persons, good ends, good rules) is back in the picture, and the moral parasite of colonialism is left alone.

Another coping mechanism of Western colonialism to normalize itself is to talk about not colonialism but the 'evolution' of yoga. Once upon a time 'yoga' meant one thing, and now it means another. But as noted in Chapter 2, this confuses changes in linguistic behaviour in the use of the word 'yoga' with changes in Yoga, as though mice have evolved because now we use the word 'mouse' for electronic pointing devices. The entirely *W*AC-ky shift from studying South Asia in terms of Philosophy to studying it in terms of Linguistics and the social sciences such as Anthropology serves to normalize the impact of colonialism in two ways. Changes in South Asia are viewed as 'evolutions' of Indigenous traditions, not colonial trauma. And the academics then are emboldened to interpret according to a *W*estern vantage, which would not be allowed if we took Philosophy seriously.

Some elementary philosophy of language is useful at this point. Philosophers of language distinguish between the literal meaning (sometimes reference) of a term and its use. The literal meaning is the systematic or basic role of an expression. And the use is derivative. Because the literal meaning of 'mother' is a female parent, we can use 'mother' in many derivative ways – for mother nature, mother superior, mother boards... The literal meaning anchors these various derivative uses. When we understand that the literal meaning of 'Yoga' where practical questions are concerned is a basic theory of *THE RIGHT OR THE GOOD*, we can then appreciate various small 'y' uses of 'yoga'. But not the other way round. If we define yoga as *āsana* practice, it will be very hard to appreciate how Yoga as taught in the *Yoga Sūtra* or the *Bhagavad Gītā* sheds any light on 'yoga' so defined.

So part of the way we know that Yoga, the philosophy, is the literal meaning of 'yoga' where questions of right action and good outcomes – questions of Yoga practice – are concerned, is to figure out the central, anchoring role of 'yoga' where practical questions are concerned. The other supportive way is to ask ourselves how we can understand 'yoga' in terms of a disagreement. This is important as it gets ourselves away from trying to use our beliefs about Yoga to understand it. And if we do the historical work of locating 'yoga' relative to a disagreement, we see that it is originally a name of a philosophical package, that is a basic view about *THE RIGHT OR THE GOOD*. Understanding 'Yoga' then is about understanding how one view called 'Yoga' is a contribution to basic questions about *THE RIGHT OR THE GOOD*.

In my research, I was the first to make the same point about 'dharma'. If we treat every use of 'dharma' as its own meaning, we multiply meanings beyond their means (violating Ockham's Razor) and we have no idea why the same word is used in so many ways. There can be no disagreement about 'dharma' then, for every use would be a solitary meaning. But if we can explicate, we can see that each perspective had its own theory of dharma, and the concept of *DHARMA* is what they were disagreeing about, which is *THE RIGHT OR THE GOOD*.

Western colonization, employing interpretation, allows people with Western beliefs to interpret everything that could be 'yoga' according to their beliefs. And the result is the idea that there are lots of different things that are yoga, and what is yoga has changed. And the key political end is to get rid of the possibility of disagreement. When we explicate, we see that Yoga is just one basic moral philosophy, and it is an option in the controversy about *THE RIGHT OR THE GOOD*. There are ways to practise this, which are small 'y' yoga. And sometimes the small 'y' yoga gets taken up by an opposing ethical theory, such as Consequentialism, as the way to pursue those distinct and contrary ethical ends.

COLONIAL TRAUMA

The *Yoga Sūtra* (YS II.3) discussion of trauma is to be found in its discussion of ignorance: *avidyā*. This ignorance, which is interpretation, leads to the creation of a false sense of self on the basis of the beliefs one employs – this is *asmitā* – and the result is happy or sad reactions on the basis of whether life fits those interpretive explanations. This is being stuck in affliction (YS II.3). What is described in the *Haṭha Yoga Pradīpikā* and subsequent 'modern yoga' fits this picture of a *kleśa* or *trauma*-based behaviour. It is a confining activity delimited to safe spaces that is treated as a refuge from the problems of life.

That Westerners flock to this picture of yoga as though it's actually Yoga (the modern version of it) speaks to the ways in which it fits with Western *saṃskāra*-s but also the colonial trauma of existing in a Westernized world. This is a world that discourages Philosophy in favour of interpretation, treats the West as the default platform for explaining everything, and then defines into privacy BIPOC traditions as religious or spiritual. And it is in this nexus of marginalization, where Yoga is supposed to be pushed into the indoor structures in gentrified parts of the world, that Yoga Studies as a version of Religious Studies typically studies yoga.

One WAC-ky example of this phenomenon is Kemetic Yoga. It is supposed to be yoga practice that originates in Egypt. According to a web page at *Yoga International*, entitled 'The Black History of Yoga'[6] (adapted from *Yoga Where You Are*[7]), 'Yoga researchers have found evidence to suggest that yoga not only originated in India but also has roots in parts of Africa, particularly Egypt.' Further, the page goes on to claim that knowledge of this practice has been suppressed owing to anti-Black racism. The idea that there was such a practice is based on postures depicted in Egyptian Hieroglyphics. The practice as described by its proponents (and this *Yoga International* page) is remarkably like what we find in the *Haṭha Yoga Pradīpikā*. Kemetic Yoga, accordingly, is about opening up channels of energy and is a practice of more steadily held postures, with an emphasis on breathing exercises and energy centres (*cakra*-s).

As we decolonize our appreciation of Yoga, the question to ask is: how did anyone come to the conclusion that Yoga came from Africa? According to the description we have familiarized ourselves with, people already had beliefs about what yoga is – beliefs consonant with 'modern yoga' – and they used these beliefs to interpret Egyptian artefacts. And on the basis of interpreting the Egyptian artefacts, they derived the conclusion that conforms to their beliefs about what yoga is and what is being depicted on the hieroglyphics. This is telling in two ways.

First, the conclusion that yoga also comes from Egypt or Africa is an interpretation, and interpretation is itself a device of colonization, central to the Western tradition. Second, the model of yoga that is employed in this interpretation is the model of 'yoga' developed under Western colonialism in South Asia. So this project of identifying Kemetic Yoga is colonizing in two ways. But it also displays and renders clear the trauma involved in this identification. The idea that Black people are not being given credit for also creating a colonial form of yoga hardly speaks to anti-Black racism. But that this is brought up in an account of Kemetic Yoga does speak to the colonial trauma of being racialized as Black in Yogaland. Modern yoga creates such a profound sense of alienation that it leads some to want to colonize African history by interpreting it according to colonial beliefs about yoga and to hence practise the African version of the West's colonially traumatized yoga. Online, this is depicted as 'Black People Reclaiming Yoga'. This phenomenon exemplifies colonialism. In colonialism, people who are thoroughly colonized repeat practices of colonialism as though that is their means of self-affirmation, and that also renders them participants in colonialism.

South Asians are also known for wanting to 'reclaim yoga' but by that is meant the 'modern yoga' of Western colonialism. That is one way to view India's efforts and success at lobbying the UN to celebrate International Yoga

Day. Addressing the UN during the opening of the 69th session of the General Assembly, India's Prime Minister, Narendra Modi, said:

> Yoga is an invaluable gift from our ancient tradition. Yoga embodies unity of mind and body, thought and action … a holistic approach [that] is valuable to our health and our well-being. Yoga is not just about exercise; it is a way to discover the sense of oneness with yourself, the world and the nature.[8]

There are certainly Aristotelian *saṃskāra*-s expressed here. Yoga is about distinguishing ourselves from nature, but for Aristotle, the good is just the natural end of a thing – unity with nature as an end is super Aristotelian! The model of oneness that is invoked resembles Neo Platonism more than South Asia's Advaita Vedānta (as noted in Chapter 3). But here too we find Yoga repackaged as a Consequentialist endeavour. We do yoga because of its great outcomes. And one of them, apparently, is oneness with everything (the very opposite of *kaivalya*). And so, International Yoga Day is marked by the practice of *āsana*.

If anyone wants to reclaim Yoga, they will have to explicate. That will lead to the discovery that 'Yoga' was a name for one unique position on *THE RIGHT OR THE GOOD* – one very important contribution to moral philosophy. If this shows up somewhere else (like Africa), under a different name, great! But this reclaiming of Yoga is a reclaiming of Yoga from Western colonialism, which prefers instead to interpret on the basis of the Western tradition. Once we reclaim Yoga, each one of us can work on our own autonomy. And in the process, we will publicly fight and agitate against colonialism via the *Yama*-s. And this will involve rejecting esoteric practices of secret powers that occur with a human teacher in hiding but disappear the moment we see the light of day. This is the Yoga of the Indian independence movement, the Yoga of the American Civil Rights Movement, the Yoga of Black Lives Matter, Direct Action Everywhere, Extinction Rebellion, the Iranian Women's protest, Indigenous people decolonizing their lives, and the bravery of Ukrainians, fighting back Russian colonization.

Of course, we can continue to practise *āsana*, *prāṇāyāma*, and other small 'y' yogas. But in reclaiming Yoga, we reclaim the practice of being devoted to Sovereignty and then practising the two aspects of it: unconservatism and self-governance. Then we can indeed celebrate Yoga publicly, but not because it provides any extra benefits (which it surely does) but because our practice of

Yoga requires that it is public. And what we achieve publicly is just ourselves: *kaivalya*.

CHAPTER 7 REFLECTIONS

- How does knowing the history of Yoga change how one views 'modern yoga'?
- How can we reclaim Yoga from the instruction of yoga?
- When you were, or if you are, a student of yoga, what kind of yoga or Yoga did you, or do you, practice?
- What is the main difference between Yoga and modern yoga?
- Yoga has benefits. What is the difference between acknowledging these benefits and adopting Consequentialism as the justification for small 'y' yoga practice?
- How does understanding history decolonially help us reject prejudices, like Islamophobia?
- If South Asians do not deserve to be colonized, as Marx and Engels suggest, what is the ethical way to consider their history?
- What are some concrete actions one can take to reclaim Yoga and ditch modern yoga?
- How does an understanding of Yoga, the philosophy, refute Singleton's view that athletic yoga *āsana* practice is not Indigenous?
- How does Yoga help us avoid the oppression of Millian and Marxist approaches to people?

CHAPTER 8

BEING AN AUTHENTIC YOGA TEACHER, STUDENT, AND PRACTITIONER

INTRODUCTION

The colonial rebranding of Yoga swaps the actual practice of Yoga with a narrow application of the practice, such as *āsana* or *prāṇāyāma*. This allows colonialism to be spared the moral and political criticism of Yoga and the decolonizing activism of Yoga. The actual practice of Yoga is the practice of a basic normative ethical theory, which is a view about the relationship of THE RIGHT OR THE GOOD. It is hence much broader than any means of practice. It is a devotion to the procedural ideal of the Right – Īśvara or Sovereignty. And this involves practising the essential traits of Sovereignty: *tapas* – unconservatism – and *svādhyāya* – self-governance. The good is just the perfection of this practice, which is our own *kaivalya* or autonomy. This is not anything extra. It is just us, but without the colonial incursion. In ancient times, Yoga the philosophy was formulated as a response to cosmic colonialism of natural influence as something that impedes and oversteps the boundaries of personal space. By the time of the *Yoga Sūtra* and the *Bhagavad Gītā*, we find awareness that this colonial intrusion also comes in the form of other people. The political version of colonialism is not a different thing so much as a different expression of the same challenge.

The relationship between actual Yoga and its various applications (small 'y' yoga) is pedagogical. When we understand what Yoga is, we can appreciate the ways in which anything we do for ourselves can be a way to practise yoga. However, if we begin with treating an application of this basic practice of Yoga as though it is the paradigm of what Yoga is, then we do not have a way to understand the philosophy, Yoga, nor why the term is used for so many different practices.

Actual Yoga practice is decolonial, as it is a practice of Devotion to Sovereignty that yields autonomy. One cannot be colonized when one is autonomous, and colonialism aims to swap Īśvara – everyone's Sovereignty – with the interpretation by way of a narrow worldview.

Actual Yoga practice is also sensitive to the conditions of trauma (*kleśa*). That is because Yoga is premised on an appreciation of the practice that takes us away from affliction. The actual practice of Yoga relies on explicatory skills to make everything explicit to preserve one's autonomy. This allows us to appreciate the implication of options and to hence have room to choose. When we do the opposite, we explain everything in terms of our perspective – interpretation – and then we do not appreciate the implications of what we are observing, nor do we have options. And in this state of having only one option, our own agency is directed to normalizing our fealty to a specific outlook.

Actual Yoga is a basic ethical theory, which is a position on the relationship between the right choice or action and good outcome. Yoga is not *every* possible view on *THE RIGHT OR THE GOOD*; it is just one option. When we practise the colonialism of anti-Yoga, we act as though the outlook we are tied to is the only option. In this state, everything has to match our expectations. This means that we cannot learn. We can only colonize.

The metaethical activity of Yoga, as opposed to anti-Yoga, recovers the space of our own agency. It facilitates this in part because it is the practice of research skills. What we find in Indology and its fashionable offspring, Yoga Studies, is the opposite of the explicatory method of research. Explication is the employment of logic to organize data, elucidate controversies, and bypass our beliefs as criteria of understanding. When we practise these basic explicatory skills of Yoga, we are autonomous as knowers. Hence, we can abide in our form and stand on our own form (YS I.3, IV.34). To explicate is to understand, for instance, that South Asians had many theories of dharma, that the disagreement among such theories was a disagreement about *THE RIGHT OR THE GOOD*, and that Yoga is just one among four basic options.

Interpretation, explanation in terms of belief, is incompatible with reason, as reasoning is about thinking, and interpretation is about our attitudes about what thought is true. And this diversion from thinking leads us to explain everything in terms of what seems true to us. This is the method of ignorance (*avidyā*) that creates a false sense of self based on those beliefs (*asmitā*) and results in the enforcing of that outlook as an intransigent affliction. Many of the isms, whether racism, sexism, or speciesism, operate according to this ignorance. Once an agent identifies with their experiences within a political hierarchy, they then conflate that political order with themselves and then use their agency to normalize their experiences. So if someone identifies with the experiences and advantages that come from being White and male in a White Supremacist and patriarchal society, then they will use their own agency to normalize this. And the result is affliction: someone who engages this choice will feel alarmed by a world of diversity and only comforted when their expectations are not challenged. In Yogaland, this same identification with the *W*estern tradition assures that there is no actual learning about Yoga. Rather, what this results in is the colonization of yoga spaces with the values and expectations of White Supremacy. There are several unobvious implications of this.

First, 'yoga' will be depicted in various *W*AC-ky ways. Instead of Yoga being a vehicle for decolonization, symbols and small 'y' yoga are redeployed to reify expectations from the *W*estern tradition. Second, practitioners will not be interested in learning. Rather, as an exercise of trauma (*kleśa*), they will reject anything that does not accord with their outlook as upsetting. Third, philosophy will seem like an irrelevant exercise. So whereas Philosophy is the basic discipline of Yoga, and our practice of Yoga is a practical application of this philosophical work, in the space of affliction, Philosophy will appear to be threatening, as it requires abandoning interpretation.

This push to interpret on the basis of the *W*estern tradition is an essential part of the colonial foundations of the *W*est, rooted in its LAT. It leads committed *W*esterners to explain everything in terms of what *W*esterners would say on the basis of their tradition, which includes their beliefs. This leads to the creation of Secularism$_2$, the idea that the default frame for public interaction, the secular, is *W*estern and everything else is religion. It leads to the interpretation of Yoga, which renders it unintelligible, as Yoga is a philosophical option, not a set of *W*estern beliefs. In colonized spaces, the unintelligibility of Yoga on the basis of *W*estern interpretation is seen as evidence of it being an esoteric and mystical process, as depicted by the colonially derived 'modern yoga'. And given the anti-Yoga method of interpretation, beliefs about yoga derived from colonized spaces are circularly used to explain yoga and to give confused people a false sense of understanding. As noted, interpretation is actually a violation of basic norms of logic and reasoning, and hence the *W*estern interpretation of Yoga is colonial as it is illogical.

In concluding our investigation of Yoga, I want to draw together the practical, action-focused implications of our investigation. I will do this, in the next section, by considering the four basic ethical theories and their responses to three challenges:

- how to learn about Yoga and to teach Yoga
- how to regulate our consumption practices
- how to find solutions to problems.

YOGA IS JUST ONE OPTION

The four basic dharma theories are each positions on *THE RIGHT OR THE GOOD*. The first three, as noted, are familiar in the *W*estern tradition and also constitute the conventional morality that the *Mahābhārata* and the *Gītā* explore as the basis of manipulation by moral parasites. Yoga is a fourth option, not known in the *W*estern tradition but nevertheless on the list of basic ethical theories, for like the other three, it accounts for the relationship of *THE RIGHT OR THE GOOD*. And, in fact, it is the mirror image of Virtue Ethics.

Virtue Ethics (the good character leads to the right choice) is the idea that the right thing to do follows from having a good character. If one lacks a good character, one has to find someone who is good and follow their lead. With respect to the question of how to learn Yoga, this is a *W*AC-ky view, as Yoga is the opposite of Virtue Ethics, but Virtue Ethics in the philosophies of Plato and Aristotle constitute very early *saṃskāra*-s of the *W*estern tradition that *W*esterners unreflectively employ. *W*AC-ky practitioners who endorse Virtue Ethics look for a good Yogi to be their teacher and regard the right thing to do as whatever they do or advise. To teach yoga, on this view, one must oneself be a good Yogi. The yoga teacher's job, on this view, is to tell yoga students what to do. With respect to consumption practices, the Virtue Ethicist will look to whomever they regard as the exemplary good person. If they eat meat, then eating meat is fine. If they are vegan or vegetarian, then we ought to follow their lead. If the Virtue Ethicist regards themselves as a good person, then they will conclude that anything they choose is fine. So it's really up to them, and their ethical choices are not answerable to others. Finally, solutions to problems are whatever a good person is inclined to do. So if one is not oneself a good person, one must find a good person and follow their direction. Hence, for instance, during the pandemic, Virtue Ethicists would look to people they admire as good people for direction on whether to mask, social distance, or get a vaccine. Of course, a lot would turn on who the Virtue Ethicist identifies as a good person. But either way, one's own interest in recovering one's own autonomy is not a basic concern for the Virtue Ethicist. So if the appointed paradigm of virtue instructed one to do something that was not in the interest of one's own independence, one would have to follow through.

Consequentialism (the good outcome justifies the right choice) is also not Yoga, so employing this as the template for learning and teaching Yoga speaks to WAC-ky *saṃskāra*-s that prize Consequentialism – a major ethical theory in the West. According to the Consequentialist, the right thing to do is what produces a good outcome, and among the right things to do, we ought to choose whatever maximizes good outcomes. So a Consequentialist has to identify an outcome they want to maximize (say happiness or the minimization of suffering) and then choose courses of action that maximize these ends. Learning 'yoga' is justified if whatever is called 'yoga' leads to those ends. Teaching 'yoga' is imparting knowledge of those skills that lead to those ends. Consumption correlatively is dictated by outcomes. And here the outcomes matter. If the outcome that the Consequentialist identifies is their own personal happiness or the avoidance of their own personal suffering, then they will consume whatever leads to those ends. They might adopt what is called an *agent neutral* outcome, like happiness as such, or the minimization of suffering as such, but they may be called to sacrifice their own happiness or suffering for the greater good. Finally, problem solving is simply about choosing the activity that gets rid of the problem. If the problem, for instance, is a pain, one would be justified in choosing a means to rid oneself of that pain even if it compromises one's autonomy. Hence, if one has a headache and this is the problem that is to be solved, and the simplest solution is deadly, this would be justified over a harder, longer process of self-care that would involve prolonging the headache and recovering one's autonomy.

Deontology (the right choice justifies good actions or omissions of actions) is the idea that while there are many good things to do (or things that are good to avoid) only some of those are justified by the right considerations. These good things to do justified by the right considerations are our duties to do, and the good things so justified to avoid are rights. Of the three ethical theories familiar in the West, and part of conventional morality, Deontology is the only *procedural* ethical theory. It prioritizes the right over the good, like Yoga. However, it defines the right in terms of candidate good things to do or avoid. Learning Yoga for the Deontologist is about learning what to do and what not to do. Teaching Yoga for the Deontologist is about teaching what to do and what not to do. Consumption is similarly regulated. Veganism, for instance, is a Deontological answer to questions of consumption. There are many good things to do in the way of consumption, but avoiding animal agriculture is especially justified, according to the vegan, because it does not support institutionalized violence (or perhaps some other reason). Solving problems for the Deontologist is just about following good practice. And it might be the case that we follow such best practices but do not solve the problem we were interested in solving. Nevertheless, we would be justified in sticking to such practices.

Yoga/Bhakti (the idea that the Right leads to or produces the Good) is the idea that the right thing to do is to be devoted to the ideal of the Right – Sovereignty/Īśvara – and the perfection of this practice (which consists of practising the essential traits of Sovereignty, namely unconservatism/*tapas* and self-governance/*svādhyāya*) is the good. One can hence correctly practise Yoga/Bhakti without being good at it, and succeeding at Yoga/Bhakti involves no extra outcomes. The good outcome is already implicit in the practice, and the practice makes it explicit. To learn Yoga, according to Yoga, requires practising Yoga. To learn Yoga is to devote oneself to Īśvara, and this involves taking on the responsibility and the problem of being independent and sovereign. Students who take this responsibility on to themselves appreciate that all of life presents opportunities to practise Yoga, and some small 'y' activities can be the focus of some pointed practice. Teaching Yoga is about sharing one's practice of Yoga with students. Teachers can then be sources of inspiration and support. But in practising Yoga, they make clear that Yoga is just one option out of many (certainly that it is just one basic option) and that learning about Yoga is a personal choice. This also involves making abundantly clear that something is a small 'y' yoga practice because it is a way to practise Yoga.

With respect to consumption practices, and all practices in Yoga, choice and activity is mediated between *tapas* (self-challenge, unconservatism) and *svādhyāya* (self-governance). In practice, we cannot content ourselves with what works for us if it is not also part of the self-governing choice we make as a practitioner of Yoga, which involves appreciating people in non-oppressive, nondiscriminatory ways. The Yogic insight into personhood as what thrives given its own unconservatism and self-governance means that we have to continually challenge ourselves to align consumption practices with the interests of people, which come in a diversity of forms, including nonhuman animals and the Earth. The obstruction to our capacity to move our consumption in the direction of what is right for people can often take two forms. First, the cost might be prohibitive. Second, the availability of such options can also be prohibitive. And this is to appreciate that there are *systemic* barriers to pro-person consumption. Hence, a fully Yogic approach to consumption would not rest with what is simply cost effective and available to ourselves (as many vegans do) but what is cost effective and available as such to any person (including wild carnivores). And this way of thinking about the challenge of consumption raises our awareness to the level of all people. This is both challenging and forgiving. For we realize that in some ways we have to contend with what we can afford and is available to us now while we agitate for systemic change – which will require addressing historical oppression and getting over anthropocentrism and the lens of our good fortune to think about others. By raising the bar and adopting a more forgiving approach to ourselves, as not part of the problem but an explanation of how things can improve, we will have to prioritize our own health, which is in the interest of all people. Put another way, as a person, what is good for us is what is good for persons. But our work as consumers is to get ourselves to understand that our consumption practices have to be part of our devotion to Īśvara, which is the shared interests of persons. For many affluent practitioners, this will require hard work to get over *saṃskāra*-s that define comfort in terms of oppressive consumption. What this work looks like, as with all Yoga, is personal but helps us all recover our autonomy.

With respect to solving problems, Yoga falls back on its basic metaethics of research. As we practise, we appreciate that we have a choice of two opposing approaches to the options. We choose the explicatory option that reveals the logic of options and their implications. Explication hence leads us to give deference to *experts* who are people who are skilled in applying explicatory methods to appreciate controversies and also thereby find answers about the controversies. This involves the *Pratyāhāra* of not being distracted by current problems and the *saṃyamaḥ* of identifying a topic (*Dhāraṇā*), exploring its implications (*Dhyāna*), and resting at the conclusion (*Samādhi*). An expert is distinct from an *authority*, which is someone who has the power to enforce an opinion. In Yogaland, authorities abound and experts are few. But taking expertise seriously is to take *research literacy* seriously. One has to practise the explicatory method of Yoga to distinguish who is a researcher and who is an opiner. As noted, in Indology and its fashionable offspring, Yoga Studies, interpretation (explanation by way of belief), the method of colonialism, abounds. The only way to know the difference between colonialism and research is to up one's research skills. That is to practise Yoga. When we practise Yoga, we appreciate options. When interpreters explain, it's just their perspective.

THE ORDINARY EXTRAORDINARINESS OF YOGA

Personally, I was reluctant to enter Yogaland to start teaching. It was my wife who prompted me to do so. She thought that students of Yoga would value my research. I thought that Yogaland was a place where no one would be interested in what I had to teach. I thought that if I instead donned a kurta and called myself 'Tantra Shyam' – entering the room with incense while regaling people with tales of my time growing up in an ashram – I would find flocks of students. And to my unsurprise, when I entered Yogaland I found lots of White people with this shtick with followers. The shtick has to do with pretending to be as South Asian as possible, via linguistic or cultural knowledge, while dangling the promise that others can join them in that exotic experience. *W*AC-ky *W*esterners love that. Because for them, given their *W*estern *saṃskāra*-s, learning Yoga is about some type of cultural immersion (Aristotle) or inclusion in a pyramid scheme with the enlightened guru at the top (Plato).

And there are certainly variants of this, like people who treat Bhakti as though it's about singing badly pronounced Sanskrit, set to nursery rhyme tunes with a harmonium, at *keertaans*! (It's *kīrtana* in Sanskrit, *kīrtan* in Hindi.) Devotion in Yogaland is recast as a group singalong experience, where no one has to work on anything, challenge themselves to learn anything, or get over their hang-ups. Basically, 'bhakti' in Yogaland is camp, retooled for adults.

What I discovered was that despite *W*AC-ky presentations of yoga, there are real practitioners of Yoga out there. When I began teaching Yoga, the philosophy, to yoga students, I found my students moved through two stages. First, the appreciation that Yoga is actually a unique option on *THE RIGHT OR THE GOOD*, and not the same as Buddhism or contrary positions. Second, the realization that Yoga, the real philosophical practice (unlike the ascetism of Buddhism, Jainism, or Advaita Vedānta), is what one does, *where* one already is, in relationship to the people that are already in one's life. As my students started to do the philosophical work of understanding what Yoga/Bhakti is, and how their actual lives are the sites for practice, almost all would report back to me that: (a) what I was teaching was life-changing (indeed, they would say that I changed their life, but it was really what I taught that did that), and (b) their relationships with other people began to improve. Unlike *W*AC-ky yoga, which is about running away and joining some new community of 'yoga' practitioners, actual historical Yoga/Bhakti is about living on one's own terms with others who you already have ties and relationships to. But as what it is to live on one's own terms is to be devoted to the same interest we all share, this self-focus turns out to also be an other-focus. As my students worked on their own personal boundaries, they also gave back to others their boundaries. The more my students stopped taking on the responsibility of living other people's lives, the more they were allowing others around them to live their own lives. And then, unlike *W*AC-ky yoga, which is an escape, like running away to join the circus, actual Devotion, actual Yoga, is about occupying the space of one's own life and allowing others to do the same. 'Bhakti' is often translated as devotion. But it is also 'love'. There can be no healthy relationships without healthy boundaries. Yoga is about recovering those dynamic boundaries.

Often, in conversation with my students, I would remark that Yoga is so ordinary. It's working on being a person, with other people around you. And so, in some ways, nothing changes and everything changes. Nothing changes as one's life is still one's life. Studying Yoga does nothing to change who your relations are, who your neighbours are, and who your colleagues are. Everything changes because now every choice is an opportunity to practise Yoga. Every interaction with others is your time to be on your own side as you interact with others, and every day provides an opportunity to shed the *saṃskāra*-s and issues that cloud one's relationship to oneself and others. And so as people practise actual Yoga, they discover themselves: the same person who was there all along but without the issues. And this discovery is a matter of self-allyship and self-friendship. As we practise Yoga, our own past is clarified. We see our past self not as a buffoon who was perpetually confused but as someone who was working on being unconservative and self-governing, as we see that self as the same self that makes our current transformation possible. Most importantly, we own our past, and our future, as real.

The political aspect of Yoga always dawns on anyone who gets to this point. For in appreciating that all of life is the site of practice is to realize that Yoga is not a retreat from the challenges of life. It is rather how we disrupt the systemic harm of our world to make room for ourselves. The apolitical nature of much of what goes on in Yogaland hence serves to highlight how it is the very opposite of Yoga and, rather, a colonial trauma response.

The struggles of activism also become easy to bear. When practising anything except Yoga, we might engage in activities for profound social change, but we do so for strategic reasons. The most obvious paradigm that facilitates this strategic approach to activism is Consequentialism. For the Consequentialist, we ought to engage in some variety of activism *as a means* to some end. But the problem is that the ends we wish, whether social justice, an end to speciesism, or the climate crisis, are not going to happen soon enough. And if the entire motivation for the life of activity is those ends, then one will burn out before accomplishing anything. But for the Yogi, activism is nothing separate from a life lived on their own terms, according to their own unconservatism and self-governance. Like the Yogi Rosa Parks who decided to sit where she chose in a bus, the Yogi engages in harm-disruptive behaviour not for any further point but to accommodate themselves. And hence, the Yogi can perpetually engage in such transformative behaviour because it accommodates them.

By practising Yoga, we also learn the metaethical value of explication as opposed to the anti-Yoga of interpretation. And with this we allow ourselves to see that the Western tradition is not the frame for everything else but rather just one tradition among many. We can hence render explicit its assumptions that give rise to a global and totalizing history of colonialism. And what we see in this tradition is that it colonizes because it is anti-Yoga – interpretive. And hence, simply practising Yoga is the easiest way to disrupt its harm of colonialism. With the practice of Yoga, the basic ethical theory, all our various interests come together in our devotion to Īśvara. *Kaivalya*, autonomy, is not an escape to anyplace else. It's just you, without the intrusion, manipulation, or confusion. And that happens because of one's willingness to engage in an ethical transformation, from a life governed by interpretation to one that is explicatory and autonomous.

CHAPTER 8 REFLECTIONS

» Are you a practitioner of Yoga or another ethical theory?

» How does adopting the logic-based practice of explication help us appreciate that Yoga is just one option?

» As Yoga practice is devotional, what changes do you have to make to be a Yoga practitioner?

» How does Yoga help one in personal relations?

» How is the decolonial activity of Yoga the same as the ordinary activity of Yoga?

» How is the idea of trauma-informed Yoga confused?

» Given that the exploratory practice of Yoga allows us to appreciate the options, is there any good reason not to practise it?

» What are the systemic barriers in your life that need to be altered to allow for pro-person consumption?

» How as a Yoga practitioner can you solve problems?

» What is your relationship to Yoga? Is it how you live your life, or is it something you regard as a part-time activity?

NOTES

CHAPTER 1

1 Daily Nous (2023) Value of Philosophy – Charts and Graphs. https://dailynous.com/value-of-philosophy/charts-and-graphs.

2 Cf. LaMonica, C. (2020) 'Colonialism.' *Oxford Bibliographies Online*. www.oxfordbibliographies.com/view/document/obo-9780199743292/obo-9780199743292-0008.xml; Butt, D. (2013) 'Colonialism and Postcolonialism.' In H. LaFollette *The International Encyclopedia of Ethics*. Malden, MA: Wiley-Blackwell.

3 Silva, G. J. (2019) 'Racism as self-love.' *Radical Philosophy Review 22*, 1: 85–112.

4 King, M. L., Jr. (1958) 'My pilgrimage to nonviolence.' The Martin Luther King, Jr. Research and Education Institute. https://kinginstitute.stanford.edu/king-papers/documents/my-pilgrimage-nonviolence.

5 For an in-depth look at this history of colonialism, see Ranganathan, S. (2022) 'Hinduism, belief and the colonial invention of religion: a before and after comparison.' *Religions 13*, 10. www.mdpi.com/2077-1444/13/10/891.

6 I write about this extensively. For one overview, see Ranganathan, S. (2022) 'Modes of Interpretation.' In W. Schweiker, D. A. Clairmont, and E. Bucar (eds) *Encyclopedia of Religious Ethics*, pp.874–886. Hoboken, NJ: Wiley Blackwell. For its impact on translation, see Ranganathan, S. (2018) 'Context and Pragmatics.' In P. Wilson and J. P. Rawling (eds) *The Routledge Handbook of Translation and Philosophy*, pp.195–208. Routledge Handbooks in Translation and Interpreting Studies. New York: Routledge.

7 See note 6.

8 For instance, see Ranganathan, S. (2016) 'Review of David Gordon White's *The Yoga Sutra of Patanjali: A Biography*.' *Philosophy East and West 66*, 3: 1043–1048.

9 See note 5.

10 See Zack, N. (2018) *Philosophy of Race: An Introduction*. London: Palgrave.

11 See James, M. (2016) 'Race.' In E. N. Zalta (ed.) *Stanford Encyclopedia of Philosophy*. http://plato.stanford.edu/archives/spr2016/entries/race.

CHAPTER 2

1 Monier-Williams, M. (1995) *A Sanskrit-English Dictionary*. Delhi: Motilal Banarsidass Publishers. Originally published Oxford: Oxford University Press 1872, enlarged 1899.

2 The Arabic verb '*nataqa*' means *to speak* or *utter*, '*mantiq*' is the word for logic, and '*natiq*' is often the word used for *rational*. (For instance, in Arabic discussions of Plato's tripartite division of the soul, the rational soul is often referred to as: *al-nafs al-natiqah*). I have

this on the good authority of Muhammad Ali Khalidi, translator and editor of *Medieval Islamic Philosophical Writings* (Khalidi, M. A. (2005) *Medieval Islamic Philosophical Writings*. Cambridge Texts in the History of Philosophy. Cambridge; New York: Cambridge University Press.)

3 For the original definition, see Ward, C. and Voas, D. (2011) 'The emergence of conspirituality.' *Journal of Contemporary Religion 26*, 1: 103–121. For a contemporary review, see Walker, J., Remski, M., and Beres, D. (2023) *Conspirituality: How New Age Conspiracy Theories Became a Public Health Threat*. Toronto: Random House of Canada.

CHAPTER 3

1 Soni, J. (2017) 'Jaina Virtue Ethics: Action and Non-Action.' In S. Ranganathan (ed.) *The Bloomsbury Research Handbook of Indian Ethics*, pp.155–176. Bloomsbury Research Handbooks in Asian Philosophy. London: Bloomsbury Academic.

CHAPTER 4

1 Gornall, A. (2014) 'How many sounds are in Pāli?' *Journal of Indian Philosophy 42*, 5: 511–550.

2 Visigalli, P. (2016) 'The Buddha's wordplays: the rhetorical function and efficacy of puns and etymologizing in the Pali canon.' *Journal of Indian Philosophy 44*, 4: 809–832.

3 De Simini, F. (2015) 'Observations on the use of quotations in Sanskrit Dharmanibandhas.' *Journal of Indian Philosophy 43*, 4/5: 601–624.

4 Truschke, A. (2012) 'Defining the other: an intellectual history of Sanskrit lexicons and grammars of Persian.' *Journal of Indian Philosophy 40*, 6: 635–668.

5 Patañjali and Bryant, E. F. (2009) *The Yoga Sūtras of Patañjali: A New Edition, Translation, and Commentary with Insights from the Traditional Commentators*. Translated by E. F. Bryant. New York: North Point Press.

6 White, D. G. (2014) 'The Yoga Sutra of Patanjali: A Biography.' In *Lives of Great Religious Books*. Princeton, NJ: Princeton University Press. See also Ranganathan, S. (2016) 'Review of David Gordon White's *The Yoga Sutra of Patanjali: A Biography*.' *Philosophy East and West 66*, 3: 1043–1048.

7 Maas, P. A. (2013) 'A Concise Historiography of Classical Yoga Philosophy.' In E. Franco (ed.) *Historiography and Periodization of Indian Philosophy*, pp.53–90. Vienna: De Nobili.

8 Ranganathan, S. (2022) 'Yoga – The Original Philosophy: De-Colonize Your Yoga Therapy (Feature Article).' *Yoga Therapy Today (Journal of IAYT)*, Winter: 32–37.

CHAPTER 5

1 Sullivan, M. B., Erb, M., Schmalzl, L., Moonaz, S. *et al.* (2018) 'Yoga therapy and polyvagal theory: the convergence of traditional wisdom and contemporary neuroscience for self-regulation and resilience.' *Frontiers in Human Neuroscience*. www.frontiersin.org/articles/10.3389/fnhum.2018.00067/full.

CHAPTER 7

1 Marx, K. and Engels, F. (1853) 'The Future Results of the British Rule in India.' *New-York Daily Tribune*, 22 July.

2 Patnaik, U. and Patnaik, P. (2016) *A Theory of Imperialism*, p.125. New York: Columbia University Press; Patnaik, U. (2017) 'Revisiting the "Drain", or Transfer from India to

Britain in the Context of Global Diffusion of Capitalism.' In *Agrarian and Other Histories: Essays for Binay Bhushan Chaudhuri*, pp.277–317. New Delhi: Tulika Books.

3 Singleton, M. (2010) *Yoga Body: The Origins of Modern Posture Practice*. New York: Oxford University Press.

4 Fenech, L. E. (1997) 'Martyrdom and the Sikh Tradition.' *Journal of the American Oriental Society 117*, 4: 623–642.

5 For more on the Far-Right Hindu departure from tradition, see Sharma, J. (2003) *Hindutva: Exploring the Idea of Hindu Nationalism*. New Delhi: Viking; Sharma, J. (2007) *Terrifying Vision: M. S. Golwalkar, the RSS, and India*. New York: Viking.

6 Bondy, D. (2023) 'The Black History of Yoga: A Short Exploration of Kemetic Yoga.' *Yoga International*. https://yogainternational.com/article/view/the-black-history-of-yoga/#:~:-text=The%20practice%20of%20yoga%20was,some%20more%20accessible%20than%20 others.

7 Bondy, D. and Heagberg, K. (2020) *Yoga Where You Are: Customize Your Practice for Your Body and Your Life*. Boulder, CO: Shambhala Publications.

8 For more on this date and the quote, see Modi, N. 'International Day of Yoga.' *United Nations*. www.un.org/en/observances/yoga-day.

Bibliography

Butt, D. (2013) 'Colonialism and Postcolonialism.' In H. LaFollette *The International Encyclopedia of Ethics*. Malden, MA: Wiley-Blackwell.

Daily Nous (2023) Value of Philosophy – Charts and Graphs. https://dailynous.com/value-of-philosophy/charts-and-graphs.

Davis, D., Jr. (2010) *The Spirit of Hindu Law*. Cambridge: Cambridge University Press.

De Smet, R. V. (1968) 'The Indian Renaissance: Hindu philosophy in English.' *International Philosophical Quarterly 8*, 1: 5–37.

Fenech, L. E. (1997) 'Martyrdom and the Sikh Tradition.' *Journal of the American Oriental Society 117*, 4: 623–642.

Hacker, P. (1995) 'Schopenhauer and Hindu Ethics.' In W. Halbfass (ed.) *Philology and Confrontation: Paul Hacker on Traditional and Modern Vedanta*, pp.273–318. Albany, NY: State University of New York Press.

Halbfass, W. (1988) *India and Europe: An Essay in Understanding*. Albany, NY: State University of New York Press. Originally published Basel; Stuttgart: Schwabe.

James, M. (2016) 'Race.' In E. N. Zalta (ed.) *Stanford Encyclopedia of Philosophy*. http://plato.stanford.edu/archives/spr2016/entries/race.

January 6th Committee (June 21 2022) Jan 6 Hearings: Full Testimony with Georgia Elections Officials. www.youtube.com/watch?v=06QUOzmMyec.

Khalidi, M. A. (2005) *Medieval Islamic Philosophical Writings*. Cambridge Texts in the History of Philosophy. Cambridge; New York: Cambridge University Press.

King, C. R. (1994) *One Language, Two Scripts: The Hindi Movement in Nineteenth Century North India*. New Delhi: Oxford University Press.

King, M. L., Jr. (1958) 'My pilgrimage to nonviolence.' The Martin Luther King, Jr. Research and Education Institute. https://kinginstitute.stanford.edu/king-papers/documents/my-pilgrimage-nonviolence.

LaMonica, C. (2020) 'Colonialism.' *Oxford Bibliographies Online*. www.oxfordbibliographies.com/view/document/obo-9780199743292/obo-9780199743292-0008.xml.

Lenski, N. (2014) 'Constantine (Classics).' *Oxford Bibliographies Online*. www.oxfordbibliographies.com/view/document/obo-9780195389661/obo-9780195389661-0127.xml.

Lorenz, H. (2009) 'Ancient Theories of Soul.' In E. N. Zalta (ed.) *The Stanford Encyclopedia of Philosophy*. https://plato.stanford.edu/archives/sum2009/entries/ancient-soul.

Lucia, A. (2018) 'Guru sex: charisma, proxemic desire, and the haptic logics of the guru-disciple relationship.' *Journal of the American Academy of Religion 86*, 4: 953–988. https://doi.org/10.1093/jaarel/lfy025.

Maas, P. A. (2013) 'A Concise Historiography of Classical Yoga Philosophy.' In E. Franco (ed.) *Historiography and Periodization of Indian Philosophy*, pp.53–90. Vienna: De Nobili.

Marx, K. and Engels, F. (1853) 'The Future Results of the British Rule in India.' *New-York Daily Tribune*, 22 July.

Matilal, B. K. (1989) 'Moral Dilemmas: Insights from the Indian Epics.' In B. K. Matilal (ed.) *Moral Dilemmas in the Mahābhārata*, pp.1–19. Shimla; Delhi: Indian Institute of Advanced Study in association with Motilal Banarsidass, Delhi.

Mills, C. W. (1997) *The Racial Contract*. Ithaca, NY; London: Cornell University Press.

Modi, N. 'International Day of Yoga.' *United Nations*. www.un.org/en/observances/yoga-day.

Monier-Williams, M. (1995) *A Sanskrit-English Dictionary*. Delhi: Motilal Banarsidass Publishers. Originally published Oxford: Oxford University Press 1872, enlarged 1899.

Oman, D. (2013) 'Defining Religion and Spirituality.' In R. F. Paloutzian and C. L. Park (eds) *Handbook of the Psychology of Religion and Spirituality*, pp.23–47. New York: Routledge.

Patañjali (2008) *Patañjali's Yoga Sūtra: Translation, Commentary and Introduction*. Translated and edited by S. Ranganathan. Delhi: Penguin Black Classics.

Patañjali and Bryant, E. F. (2009) *The Yoga Sūtras of Patañjali: A New Edition, Translation, and Commentary with Insights from the Traditional Commentators*. Translated by E. F. Bryant. New York: North Point Press.

Patnaik, U. (2017) 'Revisiting the "Drain", or Transfer from India to Britain in the Context of Global Diffusion of Capitalism.' In *Agrarian and Other Histories: Essays for Binay Bhushan Chaudhuri*, pp.277–317. New Delhi: Tulika Books.

Patnaik, U. and Patnaik, P. (2016) *A Theory of Imperialism*. New York: Columbia University Press.

Ranganathan, S. (2016) 'Kant Freedom Determinism and Obligation.' In S. Ranganathan (ed.) *Ethics 1, Philosophy*. E-PG Pathshala, University Grants Commission, Government of India.

Ranganathan, S. (2016) 'Review of David Gordon White's *The Yoga Sutra of Patanjali: A Biography*.' *Philosophy East and West* 66, 3: 1043–1048.

Ranganathan, S. (ed.) (2017) *The Bloomsbury Research Handbook of Indian Ethics*. Bloomsbury Research Handbooks in Asian Philosophy. London: Bloomsbury Academic.

Ranganathan, S. (2018) 'Context and Pragmatics.' In P. Wilson and J. P. Rawling (eds) *The Routledge Handbook of Translation and Philosophy*, pp.195–208. Routledge Handbooks in Translation and Interpreting Studies. New York: Routledge.

Ranganathan, S. (2018) *Hinduism: A Contemporary Philosophical Investigation*. New York: Routledge.

Ranganathan, S. (2018) 'Vedas and *Upaniṣads*.' In T. Angier (ed.) *The History of Evil in Antiquity 2000 B.C.E. – 450 C.E.*, pp.239–255. History of Evil. London: Routledge.

Ranganathan, S. (2021) 'Idealism and Indian Philosophy.' In J. Farris and B. P. Göcke (eds) *The Routledge Handbook of Idealism and Immaterialism*. Abingdon: Routledge.

Ranganathan, S. (2022) 'Hinduism, belief and the colonial invention of religion: a before and after comparison.' *Religions 13*, 10. www.mdpi.com/2077-1444/13/10/891.

Ranganathan, S. (2022) 'Modes of Interpretation.' In W. Schweiker, D. A. Clairmont, and E. Bucar (eds) *Encyclopedia of Religious Ethics*, pp.874–886. Hoboken, NJ: Wiley Blackwell.

Ranganathan, S. (2022) 'Yoga – The Original Philosophy: De-Colonize Your Yoga Therapy (Feature Article).' *Yoga Therapy Today (Journal of IAYT)*, Winter: 32–37.

Rawls, J. (1971) *A Theory of Justice*. Cambridge, MA: Harvard University Press.

Sharma, J. (2003) *Hindutva: Exploring the Idea of Hindu Nationalism*. New Delhi: Viking.

Sharma, J. (2007) *Terrifying Vision: M. S. Golwalkar, the RSS, and India*. New York: Viking.

Singleton, M. (2010) *Yoga Body: The Origins of Modern Posture Practice*. New York: Oxford University Press.

Solomon, R. C. (2002) *Spirituality for the Skeptic: The Thoughtful Love of Life*. New York: Oxford University Press.

Soni, J. (2017) 'Jaina Virtue Ethics: Action and Non-Action.' In S. Ranganathan (ed.) *The Bloomsbury Research Handbook of Indian Ethics*, pp.155–176. Bloomsbury Research Handbooks in Asian Philosophy. London: Bloomsbury Academic.

Sullivan, M. B., Erb, M., Schmalzl, L., Moonaz, S. *et al.* (2018) 'Yoga therapy and polyvagal theory: the convergence of traditional wisdom and contemporary neuroscience for self-regulation and resilience.' *Frontiers in Human Neuroscience*. www.frontiersin.org/articles/10.3389/fnhum.2018.00067/full.

Walker, J., Remski, M., and Beres, D. (2023) *Conspirituality: How New Age Conspiracy Theories Became a Public Health Threat*. Toronto: Random House of Canada.

Ward, C. and Voas, D. (2011) 'The emergence of conspirituality.' *Journal of Contemporary Religion 26*, 1: 103–121.

White, D. G. (2014) 'The Yoga Sutra of Patanjali: A Biography.' In *Lives of Great Religious Books*. Princeton, NJ: Princeton University Press.

Wildcroft, T. (2020) *Post-Lineage Yoga; from Guru to #Metoo*. Sheffield: Equinox.

Wildcroft, T. R. (2018) *Patterns of Authority and Practice Relationships in 'Post-Lineage Yoga'*. The Open University (PhD Thesis).

Zack, N. (2018) *Philosophy of Race: An Introduction*. London: Palgrave.

Index